THALIA:
¡RADIANTE!

Creative Director: Joanne Oriti

Library of Congress Cataloging-in-Publication Data available.

ISBN 978-0-8118-5812-0

Manufactured in China.

10 9 8 7 6 5 4 3 2 1

Chronicle Books LLC
680 Second Street
San Francisco, California 94107

www.chroniclebooks.com

THALIA: ¡RADIANTE!

Your Guide to a Fit and Fabulous Pregnancy

BY **THALIA**

WITH DR. ANDREW R. KRAMER, OB-GYN

CHRONICLE BOOKS
SAN FRANCISCO

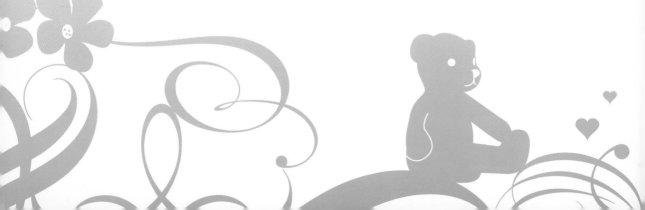

table of contents

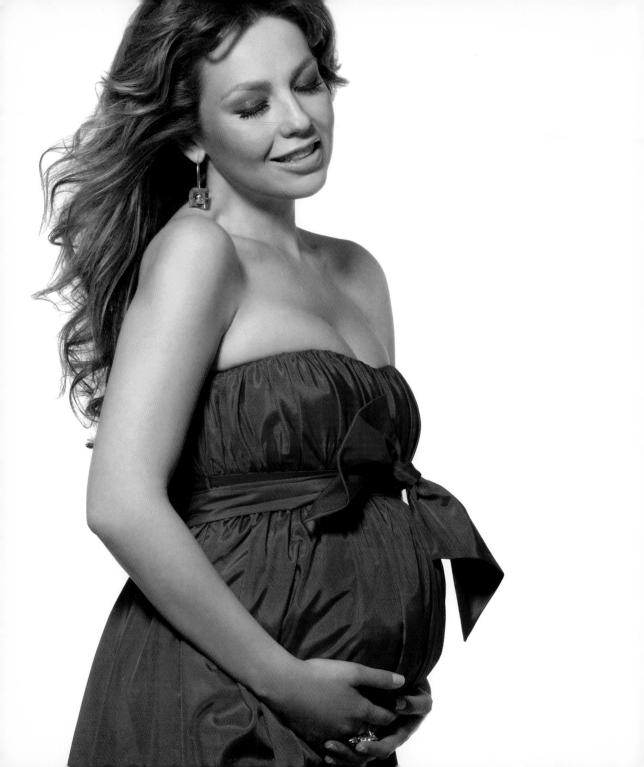

I find myself today among a new generation of mothers.

Many of us are having babies later in life, and we're not necessarily living close to our extended families. In this way, we're forced to become more independent—pioneers of our own experience and empowered by the choices we make. I wanted to write a pregnancy book from this point of view, one that would cover the basics, lend a helping hand, and, most of all, serve as a fun and informative place to come back to during what will prove to be a challenging time.

In my culture, motherhood equals queendom. Children are welcome everywhere, mothers are revered, and entire worlds of relatives circle around these women who give shape to the family and run the home. Historically, multigenerational families have always lived with one another: grandmothers helping young mothers, aunties assisting their sisters, and everyone always up for rocking a baby on their knee. Growing up among five sisters, I witnessed my fair share of pregnancies, births, diaper changes, stroller purchases, baby burpings, bathings, swaddlings,and more.

I guess it's in my genes, then, because for as long as I can remember, I've always dreamed of having a baby. Since I was a kid, I've been in love with their tiny, soft wrinkles, their sweet powdery smells, and those adorable smiles that could shatter a grown man's heart into a million pieces. And there was no shortage of babies in my household. But nothing in that world of interminable cuteness prepared me for the amazing experience of my own pregnancy.

For me, being pregnant was like living in some kind of altered dimension; everything glimmered with more brilliance, more light. All my senses became radically heightened: Sounds resonated more; colors began to pop—the blue of a clear sky became so unabashedly glorious that it felt almost piercing to my gaze. I felt less accelerated, less erratic, more balanced, and perhaps more impressionable.

But the most amazing thing about pregnancy is the way it put me in *the now* as nothing else ever had. There is just no getting around it: When you carry a baby, you are naturally forced to live in the present. You simply don't have the mental wherewithal to worry about how many oblique crunches you did at the gym that morning, or what appetizers you will be serving at your upcoming holiday party, when there is a little creature inside you who just needs for you to lie down and take a nap. When you are gestating a baby, you must defer to each moment as it comes, living each minute of each day—and living it for two. Just like that, *me* becomes *we*.

But of course, as you probably already know, it is not all smooth sailing. In the earliest weeks, my mind was swirling with emotions and questions. There was so much to address at once: doctors to choose, books to buy, questions to write down, relatives to inform, experts to consult. I felt like a tourist standing in the middle of Times Square for the first time, wide-eyed and excited but definitely a bit on edge. I was overwhelmed, and the physical impact on my body wasn't making matters any easier.

There is no shortage of books on pregnancy, but few of them spoke to me woman to woman, in the straight-up, stripped-down, vibes-up language I can relate to—which is what I needed most. And that vacancy on the bookshelves is what inspired me to write this book.

In the pages that follow you'll find tips and tidbits regarding pregnancy basics, including ideas on diet, personal style, exercise, and mental attitudes. If there is one thing I hope you take away from this book, it is this: While pregnancy is a time loaded with unknowns, it's also a time to rise up and celebrate. Yes, your body may be changing in ways that feel terrifying, but you can still look and feel gorgeous, and trimester by trimester I will do my best to show you how.

I have broken the book down into four trimesters (yes, ladies, four!), as the three months after the birth are just as crucial as the previous nine, a delicate time when both your little one and you are just beginning to cozy up to the idea of baby's life outside the womb. I offer easy tips on how to look and feel terrific through each stage of pregnancy and the postpartum period, little morsels and "fabulosity rules" that I've managed to garner from my constant orbit of stylists and makeup artists. I consulted with my own doctor, Andrew R. Kramer, MD; my pediatrician, Barbara Landreth, MD; top nutritionist Esther Blum, MS, RD, CDN, CNS; and lactation consultant Mona Gabay, MD.

There isn't enough room in this book to cover every smidgen of information about pregnancy and birth, but I've done my best to streamline things and, better still, to provide guidance, perspective, and positivity along the way. I invite you to be the guest of honor at this twelve-month celebration. It's your party (you can cry if you want to!), but I encourage you to run this show of yours with style, confidence, and grace.

straight talk

Being pregnant is the absolute mother of all highs. I'm not going to lie and say that things don't get ugly, but, before I go any further, I want to make it crystal clear that even in the darkest hours of what may seem to be hormonal chaos, there is this magnificent light that shines on you as a woman, compelling you to persist, to rise above, to endure, and to move forward with the knowledge that at the end of it all, a gorgeous little creature will look up at you with a smile on her face and a look of absolute love in her tiny little eyes.

If you are already pregnant, let me say congratulations: I welcome you to what will likely be the greatest adventure of your life, and I invite you to consider me your friend along the way. I'm no expert, but I *am* endlessly inspired by the phenomenon of creation and the power of love (the heart and soul of pregnancy), and, as a new mother, I feel inspired to share with other future mothers a bit about my own experience . . . and maybe a little simple wisdom along the way.

But all that sweet stuff aside, there is an aspect of the experience that is so raw, so unfathomable, that even your own mother, sisters, and aunts won't want to talk about it, let alone your doctor or nurse, or any magazine, book, pamphlet, or DVD. There are downright nasty things that happen to pregnant women that no one wants to discuss.

I refer to this murky realm of classified details as being guarded by The Secret Society, the mamas who keep the mysterious domain of hard-to-stomach bodily expressions on the down-low, perhaps if only to protect the mamas-to-be. My intention here is not to scare you, because the truth is that pregnancy brings with it a stronger and more intuitive you and entire worlds of magic and rapture. However, with all of that wonder and awe comes a brutal reality, ladies—one that includes unruly gassiness, endless pain, and plenty of anxiety.

Although the business of The Secret Society can be ugly, knowing the game empowers you to better handle any curveballs. More important, you quickly learn that the discomfort does in fact pass, and that even the most uncomfortable things are only minor inconveniences in the face of the profound beauty of what it really means to have baby. So, if you're a give-it-to-me-straight kind of girl, and you want to cut to the chase, take a deep breath and pour over the Dealing with Discomforts section of each chapter— you'll get your brave little self acquainted with the unspoken mysteries and tribulations of The Secret Society in no time. But try not to get too ahead of yourself. It's actually a lot more important to get your head in a positive space right now. Try to embrace this new world of yours—Babyland—floating in it freely, blissfully, allowing yourself to bask in all the excitement. You deserve it. We'll get to the challenging stuff in due time, and you'll be better off taking baby steps on your road to baby-having one moment, one feeling, and one sensation at a time.

As you move through each phase of your term and this book, it's to your advantage to keep an open mind. All kinds of things will happen to your body and brain, and the solutions oftentimes are just as baffling as the symptoms. I'll tell you this much: Never did I imagine that I'd find myself crashed out on my bed, my massive postpartum breasts covered in stinking, frozen cabbage leaves . . .

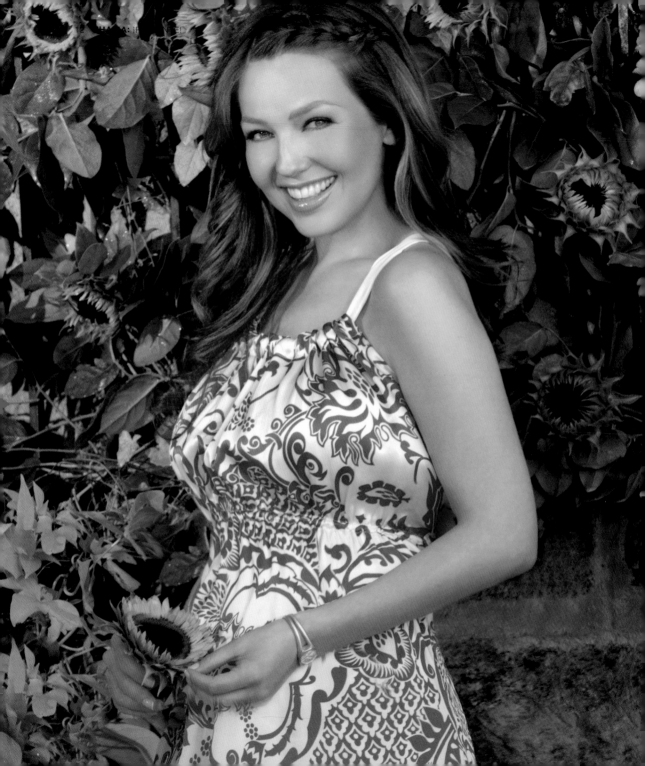

chapter 1: grown-up baby steps

FIRST TRIMESTER: WEEKS 1–13 / MONTHS 1–3

Think of your first trimester like skydiving. You simply

have to trust the mechanics of the process in order to take the leap. But to trust a process as delicate as pregnancy, you really need to embrace it. What helped me the most, and gave the most meaning to my first trimester, was to acknowledge the fact that *the early weeks of pregnancy are when the role of mother truly begins*.

The things you do for yourself during these delicate and sacred first weeks amount to your first opportunity to connect with, nourish, and love your child. Although your body may not be showing too many outward signs of pregnancy, your baby inside is growing rapidly while your body is doing the hard work of assembling the building blocks to make a healthy, happy child.

What can you expect? The reality is, ladies, pretty much *anything*: You may feel energetic or exhausted, nauseated or ravenous, elated or enraged. You might wake up happy as a clam one morning, the birds singing songs just for you, and by noon find yourself crumpled up in a corner of your bedroom praying to the gods of compassion. In my first trimester, I felt all of those feelings and sensations—and sometimes all at once. But no matter how crazy it got, my anchor of truth at every moment of distress was to remember my role as *the* one chosen to best provide for this little growing life.

With that, it is easy to understand that a smooth-sailing pregnancy begins with good prenatal care, and good prenatal care, in turn, begins with smart decision-making, a dash of daily discipline, and, above all, a positive attitude. During these early weeks, you'll be selecting your doctor, devising a birthing plan, and navigating all the options for genetic testing, never mind enduring all of the physical changes and burning questions about what lies ahead. You may feel overwhelmed—I certainly did. But that's where this book can help.

In this section I offer ways to keep your peace of mind in the midst of the juggling act. I'll guide you through what it means to be newly pregnant from a physical/developmental, mental/spiritual, nutritional, and even fashion standpoint—because even if you may not be feeling tip-top, that doesn't mean you can't still turn heads. Hopefully this chapter will answer some of your most pressing questions. But more than anything, this section helps you to prepare and strategize—and reminds you to keep your cool.

first things first

getting tested

So you think you're pregnant? It may sound obvious, but if you suspect you're pregnant then take a test! Be it a home test or in-office with a healthcare provider, there is no other way to be absolutely sure. It is critical to get tested as soon as you feel that you may be pregnant, so you can begin to take all the necessary precautions right away.

Common symptoms of pregnancy can be misleading, since they mimic symptoms of other ailments, such as hormonal imbalances, exhaustion, jet lag, a cold or flu, birth control side effects, allergic reactions, stress, food poisoning, and more. For this reason, a pregnancy test should be the first step.

Most home pregnancy tests are 90 percent accurate if you take one on the first day of your missed period, and even more accurate if you wait a bit longer. The longer you wait, the more hCG (the pregnancy hormone called human chorionic gonadotropin) you will have in your system, which is what any test, home or in-office, will detect. If you test positive at home, you should immediately see a healthcare provider for urine and/or blood tests and a subsequent complete medical exam to detect additional symptoms, such as changes in the uterus and cervix. When you find out that these professional tests are positive, let the meaning of that word resonate with you loud and clear—*POSITIVE*—and from that moment on, let it unconditionally lead your way.

And you will need all of the positive energy you can muster, because even once you know with certainty that you are pregnant, the surprises don't stop coming. For starters, you may find out a bit later in your term that you are carrying more than one baby . . . bet you never imagined *that* prospect. This can be the best news in the world to one mom-to-be and the scariest for another, but both can rest assured that there is plenty of excellent information out there on birthing twins. The book *Ready or Not . . . Here We Come! The Real Experts' Guide to the First Year with Twins*, by Elizabeth Lyons, is both sincere and extremely witty in its account of mothering twins, as is the very complete *The Everything Twins, Triplets and More Book*, by Pamela Fierro, another excellent resource.

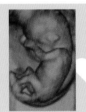

By the third month (11 weeks), your baby is 2½–3 inches long and weighs about 1 ounce.

build your dream team

There is strength in numbers—an adage that proved to be key to my birthing experience. It's essential to build a team of professionals and loved ones who will stay by your side throughout your pregnancy and delivery. Your first trimester is prime time to start thinking about who will be on your team.

Perhaps you, your partner, and your ob-gyn will be the sole members of your team. Or you might also appoint a certified nurse-midwife, who can aid in overseeing much of the prenatal, birthing, and postpartum care from a less medical, more holistic perspective. As I did, many women opt to work with a doula, a woman trained to coach you in the more emotional, nuanced aspects of your birth process, sort of like an "expert helper." After the baby is born, a lactation consultant can guide you through the process of breastfeeding, which comes easily to some women but can be more difficult for others. Once you have your team in place you can rest easy, knowing that you have a trained professional at your fingertips to answer any question you may have.

As you carefully consider the players on your team, be mindful of these considerations: How close and accessible are their offices to your home? Will your insurance cover the practice? What sort of specific or preexisting medical needs do you have that might require special attention? If English is not your first language, make sure you build a team you can communicate with well. All of these factors will matter, but most important, you should *feel* good about each of these professionals. Trust that you know what is best for yourself and what is best for your baby.

ob-gyn, oh my!

Essential in this trimester is choosing an obstetrician-gynecologist who will monitor your pregnancy. Referrals are the best way to find a doctor—or anyone on your team—especially if you and your closest friends and family are somewhat like-minded with regard to childbearing. Talk with people whom you trust—and who already have children—about positive experiences with their doctors. Another excellent referral source are physicians that you already hold in high regard. Excellent physicians usually have excellent referrals. These doctors can also match a patient's personality with an ob-gyn who would work well with that particular type of patient. In fact, I was originally referred to Dr. Kramer by my husband's internist. Then, with referrals in hand, jump on the Internet to further research doctors and facilities that you are considering. Next, try to meet with a few ob-gyns to find one you're comfortable with and one who will support any of your specific prenatal and birthing preferences.

Before you select a healthcare provider, check with your insurance company to make sure that prenatal care is covered; also verify that the ob-gyn you are considering is in your plan. If you don't have health insurance, now is the time to start sorting that out (see "The Insurance Issue," below).

The following are some basic questions that can guide your search for the right health-care practitioner:

❋ What is the proximity of the doctor's office to your home?

❋ Will the doctor accept your insurance plan?

❋ How does the doctor feel about working with a midwife and/or a doula?

❋ If you have any preexisting medical concerns, will the doctor be able to manage them, or might you also require the attention and care of someone who specializes in high-risk obstetrics?

❋ If the doctor isn't available when you go into labor, who will take his or her place?

THE INSURANCE ISSUE

Unfortunately, many women who become pregnant do not have the benefit of medical insurance. But whether or not you are insured, it's essential to get professional healthcare. There are all sorts of programs available to uninsured pregnant women, and every pregnancy can be monitored. As soon as you know that you are pregnant, see a healthcare practitioner, ask about sliding-scale costs, and look into maternity discount programs if traditional medical insurance is out of the question for you. You can also find a number of federally funded agencies and programs that assist in-need families or individuals.

GENERAL ONLINE RESOURCES

American Medical Association: www.ama-assn.org

American College of Obstetricians and Gynecologists: www.acog.org

The Society for Maternal-Fetal Medicine: www.smfm.org

American College of Nurse-Midwives: www.acnm.org

International Childbirth Education Association: www.icea.org

PRENATAL INSURANCE RESOURCES

Women, Infants and Children, a federal agency that assists low-income women: www.fns.usda.gov/wic

Medicaid, a federally funded program that helps low-income families and individuals: www.cms.hhs.gov/home/medicaid.asp

partner's part

With the whirlwind of pregnancy in full swing, it is easy to lose sight of some of the most important things. Your partner is sometimes the first to get lost in the shuffle. But they do experience the pregnancy. Consider that, to your partner, the pregnancy is essentially a testament of their love for you and perhaps the pinnacle of your relationship. The pregnancy is not only about *you and the baby* but is the incarnation of the bond between *you and your partner*. There is a tremendous built-in opportunity here to grow as a couple, as you both witness the miracle of life and human development firsthand, for the first time—*together*. In this light, your pregnancy becomes a defining moment like no other, and a profound way for you to take your relationship to a new level of maturity and strength. Agree from the outset to be open and honest about your feelings throughout the pregnancy; agree to disagree on parenting styles for now. But commit to the process of figuring it all out *together*, and let the strength of that commitment resonate throughout the pregnancy.

Not all expectant moms have partners, and many go into their pregnancy knowing full well that they will be single parents. Some are ready for that; others might be daunted. By relying on the support of friends, family, and other single moms, these women can also foster nurturing, loving, safe environments for themselves and their babies.

location, location, location

Where you give birth is as important a decision as who will assist in the birth. Some-times, though, your first choices of whom and where don't fit together, so be sure to check with your insurance company, (see "The Insurance Issue," page 19) and your doctor or midwife, to find out which hospital or birthing facility it is affiliated with. Your setting will be a big factor in how comfortable and safe you feel during the birth.

Today you can find lots of alternatives to a standard hospital birth. The most popular of these is a home birth, in which the baby comes into the world in your own living room or bedroom, away from the clinical (and some might say cold) atmosphere of a hospital. Some hospitals offer birthing rooms with a more home-like environment. These typically allow your team members—partner, mom, midwife, whomever—to be there with you and let you stay in one place for labor, delivery, and recovery instead of making the rounds from one ward to another. A few hospitals offer birthing chairs, which allow you to sit in a more upright, squatting position to help you work with gravity when pushing.

Also increasingly popular are independent birthing centers, which provide a relaxing atmosphere for births that are expected to be low risk. These are more like homes, where moms-to-be receive prenatal care and education during the pregnancy and, when the big day comes, move in with their team. With only one (or maybe two) births hap-pening at one time, the centers provide privacy and intimacy, usually even a kitchen so your partner or relatives can cook up your favorite foods. Staff is there to monitor for problems, but the general orientation is toward natural birth, so episiotomies are rare and the baby goes straight from the womb to your loving embrace. Birthing centers are associated with hospitals in case you need (or decide you want) to transfer.

Wherever you decide to give birth, assess all of your options carefully. Look at the facility's proximity to your home and accessibility to your team members (especially if your team members are not all affiliated with the location you are considering). If you decide to give birth in an independent birthing center, it is highly recommended that you also choose a hospital as a backup in case any complications arise.

BIRTHING OPTIONS

With so many birthing alternatives out there, making decisions can be tricky. Laying out the pros and cons of each option is a great way to start assessing. Once you decide on how and when to give birth, everything else can start to work around that choice.

dealing with discomforts

I spent the first four months of my pregnancy crashed out on a chaise lounge, begging the good lord to come around, cut me some slack and send some relief. If I moved even a millimeter, nausea would whack me back into immobility, putting me right down against all of my will and effort. Food was a disaster: all I could even fathom eating were

OPTION	PRO	CON
Family practitioners	They have an established relationship with you	They may not be specialized in obstetrics-gynecology
Ob-gyns	They are usually specialized	Women looking for a more natural experience might find Western obstetrics too clinical
Certified nurse-midwives	They bring a medical *and* natural approach	They may not be equipped to deal with emergencies or serious complications
Doulas	They provide sisterly comfort and support	They do not have any medical experience

crackers, bananas, and peanut butter and jelly sandwiches—and the very notion of eggs or chicken made me want to put my head in a toilet. The truth is that my life during those weeks became about resisting the urge to projectile vomit all over my house. That was it. Now, I am well aware of the fact that some women don't experience any morning sickness. And all I can say is that these are very, *very* lucky ladies. But for many of us, it's difficult to figure out what to eat, or even how to get through the day, when feeling so downright wretched. Later in this chapter I share some tips that helped me combat queasiness and some ways to look good even when you're feeling like something the cat dragged in. If you already know that you are likely to feel sluggish, I say *embrace* the fact that you have this natural built-in downtime, learn to love this (temporary) languid state, and *relax*.

But first, it is important to say a few words about what your body is going through during the first trimester. There is a lot happening, and it's best to educate yourself about what sorts of changes to expect—especially the ones you can't see. That way you won't be blindsided by the standard aches, pains, and emotional fluctuations that are normal in any pregnancy. The most effective way to cope during the first trimester is to do everything in your power to inform yourself. When you have a sense of what's coming, you can summon the strength to handle the situation. So every time you feel like throwing a chair, strangling someone, or taking a four-hour nap in the middle of a workday, take a deep breath and try to remember that whatever you're feeling is a result of your hormones in flux, muscles and joints relaxing, organs rearranging, and the weight of a little person gradually making a home in your womb. And look on the bright side: If morning sickness or exhaustion is making you as miserable as it made me, try to focus on the fact that it probably means your pregnancy is running a normal course.

In hindsight, I wish I had talked through things a bit more with my doctor or read a few more books about what to expect. I understand now, having combed through the literature on the subject, that knowledge and information are the best tools you can have to get through the toughest times. At the back of this book, I've included a list of books I found especially helpful throughout my pregnancy and recovery.

tips

Every pregnancy is different, but there are a few symptoms that the majority of us will experience in our first trimester. Here are some of the most common, plus suggestions on how to remedy the discomfort. Give these approaches a try. And at the very least, remember that for some, the first trimester is the most physically and mentally challenging. By the second trimester you should be feeling much better. Remember:

☀ **Breathlessness:** Start each day with a few deep, slow breaths. When you do feel breathless, try stretching out on your left side, which increases blood flow to the brain and can quickly alleviate shortness of breath.

☀ **Constipation:** Eat lots of fruit, especially papaya. Drink prune juice in the morning. Remember to stay hydrated by drinking lots of water throughout the day.

☀ **Cravings and aversions:** It takes a little practice, and a little trial and error, but eventually you can learn how to indulge them both in a balanced way. See "Mocktails" on page 30 for great tips on liquor-free libations, and page 38 for tips on how to have your cake and eat it, too.

☀ **Dizziness:** Try wearing an acupressure seasickness bracelet.

☀ **Fatigue:** Take various catnaps throughout the day.

☀ **Frequent urination:** A pregnant woman should always know where the nearest bathroom is located.

☀ **Gassiness and bloating:** Soak your beans for a long time before you cook them. Ease up on (or avoid altogether) cabbage, cauliflower, broccoli, and other cruciferous veggies. Consult your doctor about taking probiotics, live enzymes that are known to aid digestion and promote gastrointestinal balance. Avoid sparkling water and other carbonated drinks.

☀ **Heartburn:** Avoid spicy foods and chew your bites slowly. Antacids, such as Tums, can also be helpful and actually have two benefits. The first is that they lower the acidity of gastric acid so that when gastric acid comes up into the esophagus it is less acidic, so the heartburn is less. Tums also has absorbable calcium so it is also a great calcium supplement. Many pregnant women take antacids such as Tums to address their heartburn and also to get their daily supply of calcium.

✳ **Heightened sense of smell:** Stay out of the kitchen. Ask your partner to handle the cooking duties for a few weeks. Take a break from perfumes and heavily scented lotions.

✳ **Hemorrhoids:** Exercise regularly and eat plenty of fiber and prunes to avoid con- stipation, which can lead to hemorrhoids through straining.

✳ **Irritability:** Make sure to take time for yourself. Listen to soft, relaxing music. Meditate or sign up for a prenatal yoga class. See "Prenatal Yoga," page 50, "Hydrotherapy: Start Fresh," page 93, and "Lead with Your Heart," page 126, for additional relaxation techniques.

✳ **Larger feet:** Avoid wearing heels. Wear comfy slippers at home. Indulge in footbaths.

✳ **Nausea/vomiting:** Make sure to eat before you rise in the morning. Have crackers, dry cereal, or fruit at your bedside. Don't eat and run. Try ginger tea, candied ginger, or ginger in any form. See "The Pukes," page 45, for more remedies.

✳ **Pain in the abdomen, leg, back, and so on:** Lying down can sometimes help a bit. Yoga, deep breathing, warm baths, and meditation can ease discomfort. The only time a bath is out of the question is after you have has broken your water. You can soak for as long as you like. I like a temperature that is approximate to normal body temperature (98.6 degrees or 99 degrees Fahrenheit). No hot tubs, Jacuzzis, or saunas.

✳ **Skin changes:** Drink twice as much water as you normally drink.

✳ **Sore, tingly, and larger breasts and/or or nipples:** Employ a hands-off policy until the soreness passes.

✳ **Sweatiness and hot flashes:** Suck on ice cubes. Take cool showers.

✳ **Vaginal discharge:** Drink a glass of water or juice with one to fifteen drops of grapefruit seed extract, two to three times daily. I would also recommend wearing a thin panty liner and changing it often. Just remember that increased vaginal discharge happens to all pregnant women, and is the result of the many hormones stimulating increased vaginal secretions and increased cervical mucus production.

✳ **Water retention:** Lie on your side, not your back, when you sleep or nap. Consult your doctor about taking fast-absorbing magnesium.

Make sure to talk to your doctor about all symptoms you are experiencing to distinguish those that are cause for alarm from those that are just par for the course. There's a fine line between paranoia and precaution. If you were to call your doctor or midwife for every unpleasant, uncomfortable, or odd sensation, you'd likely be on the phone for the better part of the first trimester. So, to make your (and your doctor's) life less complicated, make sure you have a thorough discussion up front about which symptoms should receive medical attention.

healthy moms = healthy babies

The first trimester is the most important for the development of your baby. This is the crucial time when the fertilized egg is implanted in the uterus, when the embryo eventually develops into a fetus, and when the placenta begins to form and function. The placenta is created from the same sperm and egg cells and is essentially the gateway for nutrients, oxygen, and blood from you to your child. So as soon as you know you're pregnant, it's time to ditch the bad habits and behaviors that can harm your baby. Being a good mother starts right at the beginning, even when your baby is no bigger than a few rapidly dividing cells.

We all have our weaknesses, be they a cigarette, a cocktail, or a chicken-fried steak with a side of cheese fries. Trust me, it was with a heavy heart that I had to say good-bye to my martini hour to the degree that I considered sipping water from a martini glass just to get myself through the craving. But come on: giving vodka to a baby? That's just not happening in my world. As far as alcohol was concerned, I did it by the book. It was hard to accept the blatant paradox that when I was feeling the most anxious and stressed out I could no longer partake of the elixir that I knew would calm me: a martini.

Saying farewell to hot baths was no less painful for me, as my daily steaming soaks have always been sacred, my one private refuge from the rest of the world. There are many different stances on how hot is too hot when it comes to bathwater temperatures, but I chose to err on the side of caution throughout my term. I avoided the long, lingering soaks that I knew and loved and instead indulged in shorter, more tepid immersions from time to time. But the instant that I knew there was a life within me, I realized that I could no longer be nonchalant about the effects of my indulgences. I knew that one day, soon enough, I would be able to sip a martini *and* soak in a hot bath—just not for another nine months.

I truly believe that when you look deep inside yourself, you will instinctively see that the will to overcome these cravings is directly linked to that part of you that wants to nurture, love, and protect your baby. Put simply, you will crave health and wellness, and you will long for a sense of purity. The power of habits and addictions often pales in comparison to the strength of the bond that you will feel for your baby the moment you know you are pregnant. After all, this little being will be affected by every single decision you make, be it physical, emotional, psychological, or spiritual. It will experience everything with you. If you have to say farewell to your happy hour, so be it. If smoking is your thing, find a way to quit, and find it fast. If unhealthy eating is your issue, then think of this moment as the best excuse to improve your nutrition. Dare to see your pregnancy as a new beginning—not just for the family that you are creating but also for your own overall health and wellness.

In the nutrition section (see page 35), I outline what's best to eat during the first trimester. But first I want to go over the big no-nos.

smoking

While various ongoing studies debate the effects of caffeine and alcohol consumption during pregnancy, the one toxin that remains a cardinal no-no is smoking. Smoking is directly associated with miscarriages, premature delivery, stillbirth, low birth weight, and sudden infant death syndrome (SIDS). Breathing secondhand smoke isn't any better. Studies have shown that even exposure to secondhand smoke can adversely affect the placenta and possibly lead to premature birth, spontaneous abortion, and SIDS. I'm afraid there are no shortcuts here. If you're a smoker, you must make an immediate plan to quit (at the very least for the nine months of your term), and if you're not a smoker, be constantly aware of smoke around you, such as in bars or at concerts and parties. Give your baby the cleanest, freshest, smoke-free oxygen that you can breathe.

MOCKTAILS

By nutritionist Esther Blum, MS, RD, CDN, CNS. These guilt-free cocktails are especially fabulous to serve when you're hosting other pregnant friends or if you're feeling celebratory and in the mood to hear the clink of a champagne flute.

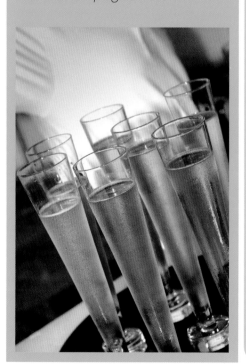

POMEGRANATE MIMOSA
(which I like to call the Mommy-granate Mimosa)

1 glass sparkling cider
½ ounce pomegranate juice
Lemon peel for garnish

Pour the sparkling cider into a champagne flute. Add the pomegranate juice. Garnish with the lemon peel or drop it right into the drink.

BABY BELLINI

2 ounces peach nectar
1 ounce fresh lemon juice
Chilled sparkling cider

Pour the peach nectar and the lemon juice into a champagne flute. Stir well. Add cider to the remainder of the glass. Stir again gently.

WINE TIME

In the mood for wine? Navarro Vineyards in Mendocino, California, makes a fantastic nonalcoholic "wine" (a grape juice, really) that did the trick for me smashingly whenever I was in the mood to raise a glass. Try the Gewürztraminer 2006 variety.

alcohol

The great alcohol debate, with its moralistic and cultural underpinnings, leaves many pregnant women in the dark. Is it, or is it not, okay to have an occasional glass of wine during pregnancy? How about half a glass? A sip of my partner's glass? If you ask a French woman, she'd probably say something like, *"Bfff! Mais ça va, tu as le droit!"* which essentially means, "Of course! You have every right!"

And for every doctor you may ask around the world, you're likely to get a different answer. European doctors more commonly condone an occasional drink throughout pregnancy. In the United States, most doctors discourage any drinking at all. For me, however, the answer was quite simple—not even a drop. And though I do love a martini as much as the next girl, after learning about the effects of fetal alcohol syndrome (FAS), I wasn't even tempted. FAS is a direct result of heavy drinking during pregnancy and results in undersize babies born with mental disorders and physical deformities who also later show behavioral, social, and learning problems. That alone was enough to stop me from reaching out when a tray of champagne passed before me. It's true that FAS is linked primarily to large and frequent intakes of alcohol, but, for me, imagining the possibility of *any* harm of *any* kind to my baby was enough to keep me resolved.

recreational drugs

Hard drugs are hard drugs, and you can't really kid yourself about the obvious adverse effects they have on you, pregnant or not. Some might argue that occasional marijuana use doesn't qualify as drug use, and they may be inclined to partake for that reason. However, marijuana use has been associated with Intrauterine Growth Restriction (IUGR) and premature births and also has been linked to neurological and behavioral problems in infants. The bottom line is that when you are pregnant, a toxin is a toxin, and no matter what story you tell yourself, your baby does not want it.

caffeine

Some studies have shown that women who drink more than five cups of coffee a day are at higher risk for birth defects and miscarriages, and for that reason most doctors agree that caffeine should be avoided during pregnancy. But many also say that minimal intake (about two cups) of coffee hardly makes any difference at all. I like to err on the side of caution when it comes to all toxins, and, frankly, caffeine isn't the best thing to have even when you're *not* pregnant. If you really savor the ritual of your morning brew, switch to decaf and drink up. Also, stay aware of some of the other major caffeine offenders, which include soft drinks, chocolate, and green and black teas. This doesn't mean you should avoid these things like the plague; just try to be mindful of how much of each you are having per day.

chemicals

Beyond what we consume, our everyday world is filled with any number of toxins, and though it's hard to be relentlessly vigilant all the time, when we're pregnant, it is our duty to try to steer clear of the kinds of chemicals that can be harmful to the fetus. Lead, for example, which can be found in water, is known to be dangerous for the neurological development of a fetus. So make sure the water you drink is lead-free. Some faucet water filters will remove lead and other pollutants. For the most part, lead is no longer used in most American paints, but if you live overseas, or in an old house or building, you might want to look into it.

Your everyday household cleaning products may contain toxins, so try not to inhale them or handle them directly. Wear rubber gloves when you clean, and switch to pump sprays instead of aerosols. Definitely stay away from the stronger products, such as oven cleaners, whose chemicals are intensely toxic. Or go green—it's good for the environment, and it's good for your baby.

activities to avoid

Just as there are certain substances you should be avoiding, there are also some activities that may have harmful effects. For the nine months of your term, you should consider putting on hold the use of hot tubs and saunas, for example. Most ob-gyns will tell you they are absolutely off-limits, as a pregnant woman's body temperature should not exceed 102 degrees Fahrenheit for more than ten minutes. Heating blankets are a no-no for the same reason, as they tend to elevate the body temperature too quickly.

Be mindful of your microwave usage, because even though most research shows that microwave exposure is safe, it is also known that fetuses are vulnerable to the kind of heat generated by its waves. If you use a microwave oven, try not to stand directly in front of it when it is on, and make sure it is not leaking.

Another heat-related activity to avoid is tanning, though not necessarily because of the heat itself. As you will likely notice even before you hit the beach, pregnancy can bring on some unusual skin discoloration, which will only be aggravated by the sun. If you're a sun bunny and just can't live without your regular dose of sunshine, use a good sunblock with a sun protection factor (SPF) of at least 30.

Speaking of rays, there are differing opinions about the safety of X-rays during pregnancy, but again, you should err on the side of caution. If your dentist proposes a series of elective X-rays, it's probably best to turn them down unless your dentist thinks they are absolutely necessary for proper dental care. In these circumstances your dentist should use a lead apron to shield the abdomen and pelvis. This will protect these areas, and your baby from exposure to radiation.

miscarriage and misconceptions

If you are a first-time mom, or if you've had a history of miscarriages, you're likely to feel some anxiety about the possibility of a sudden, unexplained end to your pregnancy. This is totally normal—in fact, it's part of the deal during the first few months of pregnancy. The anxiety is understandable, since early miscarriage occurs in about 10 to 20 percent of recognized pregnancies. If we include unrecognized ones, the statistic may be even higher, since most miscarriages happen in the first three weeks, before a woman even knows that she's pregnant. Research shows that 70 percent of first-trimester miscarriages result from chromosomal abnormalities that lead to anembryonic pregnancies, in which the fertilized egg attaches to the uterine wall but only the pregnancy sac develops, without the embryo. In most cases the exact cause is a chromosomal abnormality that is not compatible with continued development, though there is no evidence that a tendency to miscarry is hereditary. So if it happens to you, it is likely a very low probability event. There is a statistical probability to miscarrying that is based on a woman's age: the probability of miscarrying increases as a woman gets older just like the probability of Down's Syndrome increases as a woman gets older. Down's Syndrome just happens to be a chromosomal abnormality that is capable of "surviving" the first trimester. Other chromosomal abnormalities (like an extra chromosome 3) always will end in a miscarriage. The good news is that if it happens to you, the likelihood is that the next time it won't (a one in four chance of miscarrying, for example, also means a three-quarter chance of not miscarrying). So if it happens to you, it could very well be a random event.

Certain risk factors—such as hormonal problems, chronic health issues, infections, high fevers, accidents or injuries, and age—*may* contribute to the chance of miscarriage, although you should not automatically assume that you are destined to miscarry if any of these pertain to you, especially since most health issues today are treatable and manageable. However, there are other things—like smoking, heavy drinking, using street drugs, exposure to large doses of radiation, or having an intrauterine device (IUD) in place at the time of conception—that are known causes of miscarriage, so you should work hard to avoid them. Finally, there are factors that may be beyond your control: if you naturally have a malformed uterus or large uterine fibroids, for example, you may be at a higher risk for miscarriage. Again, however, many of these complications have solutions, thanks to new advances in medicine.

Women typically start worrying when they see spotting or feel a strange cramp or pain—yet these are totally normal for pregnant women. The staining can happen because a woman's cervix is more vascular and bleeds easily. The uterus is enlarging and ligaments that support it are stretching.

With a calm mind and a watchful eye, you should monitor any spotting or pain, especially if you have a history of miscarriage. If the pain is severe or persists, or if you bleed as if you were menstruating or heavier, you should immediately call your doctor. If you must, go to the emergency room, but make sure you contact your doctor first and if possible leave a number, such as a cell phone, where he/she can reach you. Generally speaking, it is always a good idea to call and touch base with your doctor (sooner rather than later) if you notice staining or bleeding.

table for two: what to eat in the first trimester

I'd say that I maintain a pretty balanced diet. I stay in shape, I eat right, and I drink a lot of water. But once I became pregnant I realized that I had no idea what I should or shouldn't be eating for the development of the *baby*. Should I cut out red meat? Eat more fish? Less fish? What's wrong with broccoli? Is sushi really off-limits?

After many conversations with my doctor and lots of reading and cross-referencing, what I learned about eating right during pregnancy is really not that complicated: Eat whole foods, colorful foods, and varieties of foods. Eat meals that are high in protein and low in refined carbs. Eat organic produce. Consume small, frequent meals. Drink lots of water. Sticking to high-nutrient, low-fat foods, green leafy vegetables, lean protein, and fresh fruit is the best approach to a clean, balanced, well-fortified diet—and it also happens to be the recipe for a perfect pregnancy diet.

But if you are one of those people who simply does not understand a world without sugar, or if you never jumped on the whole-grain bandwagon, or if you just can't be spoken to until you've downed your double latte in the morning, I sincerely encourage you to take a good, long look inside and force your large-living self to up and change. Never in your entire life has it mattered more, *because this time it is for your baby*. This mantra should give you the strength to make a serious commitment to eating well and avoiding anything risky. As a friend of mine likes to say, "Nobody ever died from not eating sushi."

Think of your pregnancy as an opportunity to reconfigure your relationship to food and eating, a way to clean the slate and reestablish your diet on a foundation of fresh, whole foods and plenty of water. Use this special time to discover new healthy recipes. Get them from friends, scour the Internet, comb through cookbooks—make it your mission to find healthy meals that will be good for you and your growing family both during and beyond the pregnancy. One of the great things about this moment in your life is that your body somehow knows what it needs, and at the same time it is repelled by the things it knows it should not have.

But eating well can be tricky, especially during the first trimester. It definitely was for me. I'd wake up quite literally dry-heaving at the prospect of that dollop of cottage cheese I was planning to add to my ruby red grapefruit for breakfast. I kid you not—there were

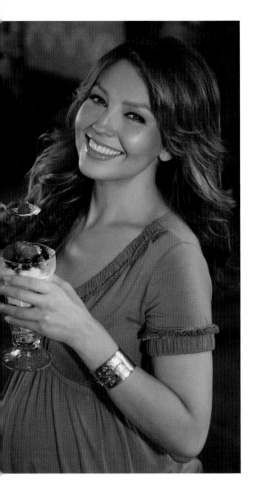

times during my pregnancy when water itself seemed like the enemy. But the moment would pass, and the next thing I knew, I was craving a giant pile of fresh arugula and diced avocado with lemon juice, olive oil, and fresh Parmesan cheese—which turns out to be a gloriously perfect meal choice. It always helps to remember that no matter how nauseated you may feel, this sensation will die down, and you will eventually want to eat. (Read on for tips and menu suggestions on how to quell the quease.)

supplements

One thing you will have to get used to (unless you are already a veteran vitamin-popper) is what I call the *daily handful*, otherwise known as prenatal supplements. Typically, your ob-gyn will prescribe a cocktail of vitamins and minerals such as folic acid, calcium, vitamins A, C, D, B6, E, zinc, copper, and iron. There are variations on the combo, depending on what your doctor decides suits your particular needs.

Because I felt nauseated all the time and couldn't eat much, I became anemic, so my doctor gave me iron supplements. (These made me constipated, so I had to take a stool softener as well . . . but more on that later.) The calcium pills were also hard for me to take, because during my first trimester nothing seemed to get past the nausea, not even a pill. My doctor, ever the clever one, gave me the calcium in the form of caramel and chocolate chews, which tasted great and felt more like special treats than vitamin tablets. Also, if you have acid reflux, which many women experience during pregnancy,

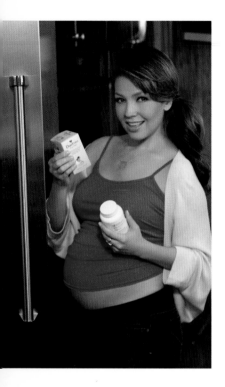

Tums not only relieves it but also serves as an excellent source of calcium. Make sure to ask your doctor what's best for you.

While the daily handful will arm you with necessary nutrients, don't kid yourself into thinking this affords you the freedom to start gorging on Krispy Kremes and pork chops. Supplements are not a free pass to chow down on whatever you want—in fact, one of the most important things you can do for yourself during your pregnancy is aim to get your vitamins from whole foods. Supplements are called "supplements" for a reason. Use both the supplements and your diet to give your baby exactly what a growing body needs. The bottom line is that eating right and downing that daily handful is the first act of true love and respect that you can give to your child.

having your cake and eating it, too

For all the foods I thought I could never live without, I found lots of healthy and delicious alternatives. Simple substitutions afforded me the opportunity to be a healthier eater *and* get creative with my menus. Consider the savvy advice of Esther Blum, an award-winning nutritionist who wrote a fantastic book called *Eat, Drink, and Be Gorgeous.* As Blum advises, simple things like switching from regular pasta to soba (buckwheat) noodles, or going from chocolate ice cream to chocolate sorbet can make a big difference. Soba is a terrific source of fiber, and sorbet has little or no saturated fat, whereas ice cream is loaded with it. With a little resourceful thinking, I could give in to my cravings without doing damage to my diet. Instead of mashed potatoes, I'd make

THE DON'T-EVEN-THINK-ABOUT-IT LIST

Here's a handy list of what you really can't have and why you really can't have it:

Because it's crawling with bacteria:

❋ Anything showing mold. You might also want to avoid certain cheeses like Roquefort or Camembert, which are manufactured with mold.

❋ Rare or raw meat

❋ Any raw vegetable, such as sprouts, pulled from or off the ground is filled with bacteria often coming from the waste products of other animals. Lettuce also could be included. These are not absolute "no-no's" but raw vegetables need to be washed very carefully and thoroughly.

Because of the risk of listeriosis, a disease caused by bacteria that can cross into the placenta and affect fetal development:

❋ Cold cuts

❋ Hot dogs

❋ Raw or undercooked meat

❋ Raw, undercooked, or smoked fish (this means sushi)

❋ Unpasteurized dairy products, such as raw milk or soft cheeses (unless they are made with pasteurized milk)

Because of the risk of salmonella, a disease caused by bacteria:

❋ Raw or undercooked eggs

❋ Raw or undercooked poultry

Because it impairs fetal development and could have long-term impacts:

❋ Alcohol

❋ Certain medications (ask your doctor to assess any medicine you take, whether prescribed or over-the-counter)

❋ Exposure to lead in water and in paint dust or fumes

❋ Liquid paints and solvents (water-based soluable paints are considered ok).

❋ Nonstick and stain-resistant products

❋ PCBs or industrial chemicals

❋ Pesticides and herbicides

❋ Recreational drugs

Because these fish contain high levels of mercury that can be harmful to the fetus:

❋ Grouper

❋ Mackerel

❋ Mahimahi

❋ Shark

❋ Swordfish

❋ Tilefish

❋ Tuna

Because not enough studies have been done for us to know the effects of the chemicals used:

❋ Antidepressants that are selective serotonin reuptake inhibitors, or SSRIs

❋ Cosmetics that have phthalates, parabens, or methylisothiazolinone

❋ Hair dye and highlights, except for pure henna

❋ Over-the-counter sleeping pills

❋ Whitening products for the teeth

Because even though herbs are natural, they have not been sufficiently studied for us to know their long-term effects:

❋ Strongly caffeinated teas, including black tea and green tea

❋ Certain common herbs: comfrey, cascara, echinacea, goldenseal, mugwort, mandrake, pennyroyal, rue, wormseed, wormwood

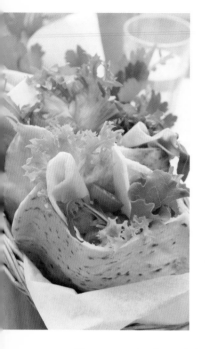

mashed cauliflower or parsnips; I switched from sweetened frozen yogurt to plain yogurt with a sprinkle of brown sugar or a drizzle of honey; instead of using bread for my sandwiches, I wrapped everything in lettuce, such as chicken with avocado, and mozzarella cheese with tomato slices. For dessert, I would sauté mixed berries—strawberries, blackberries, and blueberries—and eat them with a dollop of plain nonfat yogurt. It's a perfectly fresh fix for a sweet tooth.

Now, I understand that busy moms-to-be often don't have the time to prepare labor-intensive meals. I also know that the prospect of spending time in the kitchen is pretty daunting to most pregnant women, what with the onslaught of aromas all swirling together, practically attacking the senses. But that does not mean you should head for the frozen-foods aisle. There are simple, quick things you can prepare. One of my favorite snacks to make was fresh vegetable juice. It's fast and easy. Best of all, green leafy vegetables are packed with vitamins and minerals. Wash thoroughly and juice them fresh (nausea permitting) for a fantastic way to get the goods directly—and quickly—into your system. Soup is also great for providing multiple nutrient sources in one quick meal—plus, you can make large amounts of it and eat the leftovers for the next few days.

Most doctors recommend three servings of protein daily for pregnant women, or at least 75 grams every day, because the amino acids in protein are the foundation of human tissue. Frequent protein intake helps prevent complications and fortifies your baby with the fundamental building blocks for physical and neurological development. Amino acids are the basic elements of human cells, and since your baby's cells are dividing so fast, your amino acid intake needs to be consistent and constant.

Lean protein such as sliced turkey breast, turkey burgers, grilled chicken, and cooked fish are perfect, as are egg whites, cottage cheese, and whole grain breads, pastas, and cereals. If seafood is your thing, choose wild Alaskan salmon and halibut, which are low in mercury. Vegetarians can get plenty of protein from soy-based products. Lionesses out there, you can have your steak, just be extra certain that it is cooked through.

eating well

Conventional fruits and vegetables are typically sprayed with pesticides and herbicides, which may cross through the placenta to the baby, so many expectant mothers are inclined to eat only organic produce. This is not a bad way to go, if you can afford it. Regardless, all fruits and vegetables should be thoroughly washed. If you can only afford to go partially organic, here's a list of foods you might want to spend that extra buck on:

❋ Meat, poultry, and eggs

❋ Dairy products

❋ Fruits such as strawberries, red raspberries, cherries, imported grapes, nectarines, peaches, apples, and pears

❋ Veggies such as bell peppers, potatoes, and spinach

Eating well when we're eating for two is also tricky because we might be inclined to cut ourselves a bit too much slack and eat as if it were an Olympic sport, almost proud of indulgences. Taking these sorts of liberties is *not* what good prenatal care is about. Granted, listening to your body for cravings is an important intuitive tool for your (and your baby's) nutrition, but when you find yourself downing a pint of ice cream nightly simply because you feel like it, you will unquestionably gain unnecessary weight. This is counterproductive and possibly even detrimental to the pregnancy and birth.

Every woman should consult her own doctor about how much weight she should gain, but the one thing to keep in mind is that if you're looking for an easy delivery, *size does matter*. The larger you get, the less flexible and more clumsy you become, two things you most definitely do not want to be as you make your way into the delivery room or birthing room.

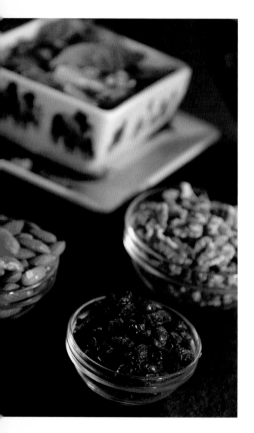

Daily exercise and eating right are cornerstones of a solid prenatal regimen. In general, most doctors recommend that you gain no more than 10 pounds during the first trimester of your pregnancy; 12 to 14 during your second trimester; and 8 to 10 pounds in the third trimester. Most doctors usually recommend that you gain a total of 25 to 35 pounds for the entire pregnancy. Just remember, everything you eat (both quality and quantity) directly affects your baby's organ and brain development, and your baby's birth weight.

All of a sudden that pile of cheese fries isn't just about cellulite anymore! Remember, to keep weight gain in line:

❋ Keep saturated-fats intake low

❋ Eat unrefined sugars, breads, and pastas

❋ Keep your protein clean and lean

❋ Sip water all day

Fruits and vegetables are great, of course, but as we know, much of the produce we consume is loaded with contaminants like pesticides—which we should try to avoid, especially when we are eating for two. It helps to know which products are most contaminated and which are the least. According to nutritionist Esther Blum and the Environmental Working Group, here is the breakdown:

12 Most Contaminated	12 Least Contaminated
Apples	Asparagus
Bell peppers	Avocados
Celery	Bananas
Cherries	Broccoli
Imported grapes	Cauliflower
Nectarines	Kiwi
Peaches	Mangoes
Pears	Onions
Potatoes	Papaya
Red raspberries	Pineapple
Spinach	Sweet corn
Strawberries	Sweet peas

Washing produce gets rid of a lot of the toxins, but some pesticide residue can make its way into the fruit or vegetable's skin. However, peeling the skin strips away all of the best nutrients. So the best thing to do, if you can, is to eat as much organic produce as possible, especially when it comes to foods in the left-hand column.

EATING AT A GLANCE

If you're pressed for time (and who isn't?), keep this list handy while you shop and prepare meals to get the most out of healthy eating:

* Avoid caffeine (for once in your life, come on)
* Avoid MSG (monosodium glutamate), as it can cause allergic reactions
* Avoid processed foods
* Buy organic produce
* Consult your doctor or midwife about which herbs are okay for you
* Drink fresh juice
* Drink lots of water
* Eat a variety of foods
* Eat naturally colorful foods
* Eat small meals throughout the day
* Use your blender or juicer (or get one)
* Wash your hands thoroughly before cooking
* Wash produce well

on the go and guilt-free

If you don't have time to go all out for your meals, there are plenty of great snacks that are not only healthy but also totally portable. These are the quick little munchies you can snack on throughout the day, which is essential when you are pregnant, because it keeps your blood sugar stable:

* Blueberries and other berries
* Carrot and celery sticks
* Grapes, plums, peaches, and apples
* Low-fat popcorn
* Olives
* Roasted almonds, other tree nuts, and seeds
* Sesame rice crackers
* Soy crisps
* String cheese

Remember that breakfast is the most important meal of the day, fueling you (and baby) with the day's first round of nutrients and kick-starting your metabolism into gear. Be diligent about breakfast. If you don't have the energy or time to make a huge production of it, have some of these:

✳ Banana

✳ Breakfast bar

✳ Hard-boiled egg (you can boil a half dozen at a time and store them in the fridge)

✳ Instant oatmeal

✳ Whole grain toast with a slice of cheese

✳ Yogurt or protein beverage

the pukes

I'm not going to even grace this wretched state by calling it "morning sickness," because (a) everybody knows it lasts way past morning, and (b) for me it seemed to always culminate in a riled-up, sweaty, dizzying series of, well . . . pukes. Not pretty, but very real, and essentially what I spent my first thirteen weeks grappling with. This is a classic first-trimester state of affairs, and although it can be challenging, understanding why all this is happening in your body undeniably helps you overcome it.

Rapidly changing hormone levels stimulate a part of the hypothalamus in the brain that is known as the chemoreceptor trigger zone (CTZ); this region of the brain once stimulated is responsible for causing nausea. It is generally believed to be the result of hormone levels changing in your body as well as the drop in your glucose levels as your body works to create life. It is also said that nausea and vomiting during the first trimester is actually beneficial, somehow protecting the pregnancy. Your interminable nausea, in a sense, is

TAMING THE BEAST

Here are my personal favorite remedies for combating nausea:

* ❋ Cinnamon gum (never mint)
* ❋ Cheerios and Lucky Charms (no joke, they did wonders for me)
* ❋ Fruit Popsicles
* ❋ Matzo ball soup
* ❋ Sour-apple candies or lollipops
* ❋ Sparkling water with lime and salt, which in Mexico we call *sueritos*
* ❋ Wasa crackers

warding off anything that may be harmful or even off-putting to your baby. (Raw chicken, for example, which is crawling with bacteria, is a common aversion for women during pregnancy.) It really is another one of those miraculous built-in systems of protection.

And for those really horrid moments when the nausea just grabs you by the hips and sits you right down, I cannot say enough about the age-old, tried-and-true antidote of ginger, be it made into a tea or chewed on directly. Throughout history, ginger has come to the rescue, assuaging nausea for many a mama-to-be.

When you honor what is going on in your body, it is much easier to accept and endure the pukes. See it as a sort of testament to the beautiful ferment happening inside, the juices of creation gurgling in its vessel . . . *you.* And if that fails, take a few really deep breaths and gently remind yourself that every moment of discomfort eventually does pass.

My best advice for beating nausea is not overstuffing yourself, staying well hydrated and nourished, and snacking on foods that will keep your motor running and your quease barometer balanced. Other foods that have been known to tame nausea are lemons, wild yam root, which can be taken as a supplement, and papaya, which can also be taken in pill form if the smell is too strong for you. Vitamins B5 and B6 can also help ease morning sickness. Consult your doctor about dosage.

ease the quease

According to Esther Blum, "Nausea may be controlled, lessened, and occasionally elimi-
nated. While no single idea helps all women, sometimes it is a combination of many
that work well together." Try some or all of the following to see what works best for you:

1. At night, place dry toast or dry cereal at your bedside, along with jam or jelly. In
the morning, before rising, eat these slowly. Stay in bed for fifteen to twenty minutes;
then get up slowly (without making any quick movements), and avoid unnecessary
bending while dressing. Allow ample time for dressing, eating, morning chores, and
getting to work. Avoid rushing.

2. Eat only solid foods early in the day, and don't gulp down any fluids. Take small sips
of water. Divide breakfast into two or three small snacks to be eaten at one-hour intervals. Consume cooked fruit or well-ripened bananas. Avoid fried or fatty foods. Later on,
if thirsty, suck on ice cubes or sip clear, sweetened tea, coffee, or skim milk.

3. Chew food well and eat slowly. Keep portion sizes small. Choose foods that you
really enjoy to ensure a pleasant meal.

4. If certain food odors are bothersome, omit these foods. Fumes from open-pot cooking, frying, or coffee brewing may cause nausea. Use the oven, cover pots, and make
instant (decaf) coffee.

5. Avoid fat, oil, and mayonnaise. Trim fat from meat before cooking, and use very little
salad dressing. Don't add much butter to cooked food. Use no gravy or cream sauces.
Bake, broil, simmer, or stew meats.

And when you finally *do* feel like eating, follow your instincts and eat what seems most
appetizing. Pay attention to your nose, since it will be in its most sensitive state, and let
it dictate what seems to be the best or worst things to eat. Be patient with yourself

and trust your gut, but also stock your kitchen with the right foods from the get-go so that you have a solid foundation of ingredients to work with (see Table for Two, page 35).

So remember these tips to combat morning sickness:

❋ Nibble on dry crackers

❋ Sip ginger tea or chew on ginger candies

❋ Sip homemade vegetable broth or matzo ball soup

exercise and the art of body-rocking

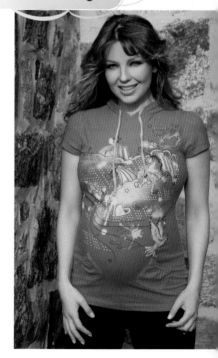

During my first trimester, the last thing in the world I wanted to do was exercise. I felt utterly exhausted and I had the pukes. It was all I could do to drag myself out of bed each morning. But I knew that if I didn't get moving, I would just feel worse. I also knew that by being active, I would be doing the baby and myself a fantastic service, giving the priceless gifts of improved circulation, metabolism, strength, and flexibility. So I made a point of spending at least twenty minutes a day exercising. Even if it was slow, gentle yoga, I made sure I got my body moving and my blood flowing.

The beauty of exercise is that it's just as good for your mind as it is for your body—it also benefits mood and energy levels. Any fitness routine you put your body on now will come in handy when you are carrying, and later delivering, a baby, because you will be that much more limber, strong, and peppy. In fact, a solid exercise regimen throughout your term is pretty much guaranteed to make the entire experience easier. Regular exercise means you'll have less weight gain, you'll recover faster from the bodily stress of pregnancy and childbirth, and you'll be stronger for the delivery itself.

In your first trimester, exercise will relieve swelling, water retention, aches, morning sickness, and pains, and it will help you sleep better. A lot of women feel more energized after some light exercise or yoga, so this may help you combat exhaustion and fatigue. In the same way that you are opening your mind about what you eat, consider your pregnancy a time to open your mind to new forms of exercise.

Before starting any exercise regimen, be sure to check with your doctor. Most doctors generally discourage high-impact exercise, and there are some yoga poses that you should avoid. Something you *can* do is to indulge in a prenatal massage, which is a lovely treat that is great for circulation, tension release, pain relief and peace of mind. Also, if you are too tired during the first trimester (or second or third), prenatal massage might be a nice and healthy luxury that will at least get the blood flowing.

SHAKE IT, BUT DON'T BREAK IT

The following are activities and postures you should avoid:

❇ Any sport that risks injuries from falls, such as horseback riding, skiing, or snowboarding

❇ Bikram yoga (or yoga in heated rooms)

❇ Certain yoga positions involving twists, jumps, rapid inhales, inversions, back bending, abdominal work, and lying on the belly

❇ Heavy lifting

❇ Tennis, particularly doubles, is generally okay, however racquetball and squash may be a little too intense.

Your doctor can tell you which exercises are okay for you and how hard you should push yourself. You will find an entire world of fantastic exercise programs tailored for pregnant women available on DVDs, in books, at your gym, online, and through your other pregnant friends. See the resources section at the back of this book for a list.

the super vagina

One of the most beneficial exercises for pregnancy is something you can do anywhere, anytime. It's a set of exercises called Kegels, consisting of simply contracting and releasing your vaginal muscles. (Wink, no one has to know.) These exercises strengthen the muscles of the pelvic floor, which are essential players during delivery. These exercises are also excellent to continue postpartum. They keep things, how shall we say, *firm*.

Generally speaking, it's best to designate a set time each day to practice anything, but the beauty of Kegels is that you can do them anytime you want, anywhere you want. To perform Kegels properly, contract your pelvic floor muscles, which most of us recognize as that distinct squeezing sensation we feel when we try to prevent the flow of urine. It's the vagina muscle. Don't get too complicated with it. Just squeeze. You instinctively know what it is. Squeeze in ten-second intervals for sets of at least ten, and incrementally increase the number of reps and sets as you continue to build strength. Your body (and especially your nether-petals) will thank you.

prenatal yoga

For me, prenatal yoga proved to be one-stop shopping for fitness and peace of mind. Here was an hour every day of my term when I was able to not only enter a deep state of relaxation but also to stretch my tired body—releasing tension and simultaneously

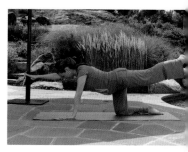

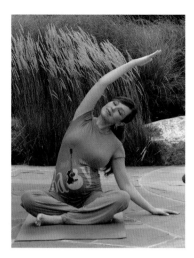 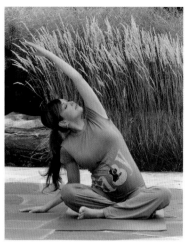

strengthening key muscle groups that I would later use for delivery. Union of mind and body, indeed. Prenatal yoga was my saving grace because it covered all bases: It has deep physical and mental benefits that affect you and your baby in an almost poetic way.

Prenatal yoga is different from regular yoga because it aids in relieving the common discomforts your pregnant body experiences,and it also encourages you to look within yourself to try to align physically, emotionally, and mentally with the prospect of child birthing. It's a sacred time when you disengage from nagging little worries and free up the physical tension that comes with your changing body.

I believe the key to a great prenatal yoga regimen is to find a teacher you like a lot, or feel comfortable with. There's nothing like a really inspiring yoga teacher to fuel your motivation, and when you find the right person, don't be afraid to ask questions about how often you should be practicing or what postures you should be avoiding, given your circumstances. Again, as with all forms of exercise, women should check in with their doctors before starting

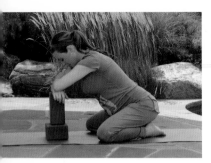 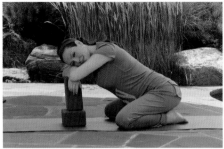 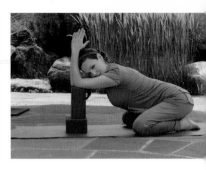

prenatal yoga. Also, be sure to tell your yoga instructor that you are pregnant, even if you are keeping it from everyone else in the world.

Now, not everyone has the luxury to spend the time and money on these types of classes. Not to worry: There are dozens of books and DVDs out there that can also guide you through the postures. However, be sure to discuss all of the poses with your doctor to ensure that they are safe for you. Two fantastic DVDs I recommend are *Prenatal Yoga with Shiva Rea*, taught by a preeminent, world-renowned yoga instructor, and *Yoga Pregnancy* with Heather Seiniger, a certified prenatal yoga teacher and mom. One of the books that most inspired me, and not just for its yogic teachings, was *Bountiful, Beautiful, Blissful* by Gurmukh Kaur Khalsa, which guides you through your pregnancy as a holistic fusion of body, mind, and soul. It is chock-full of meditations, visualizations, mantras, and postures that aim to help you through your pregnancy.

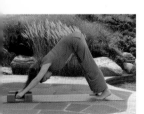 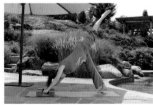 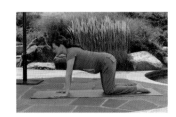 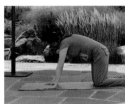

work it wherever, whenever

In general, the more exercise you do while you are pregnant, the more quickly you will be able to shed your baby weight and return to your sexy self postpartum. If you have never been much of a workout girl, now is the perfect time to start. I am not suggesting you have to reinvent yourself as a fitness bunny. You don't have to be too ambitious. Start small: Walk to work (if it is realistic) instead of taking the car. Park far from the entrance to the mall. Take the stairs instead of the elevator. Do three sets of wall push-ups and leg lifts at least three times per week. Fuel your determination by reminding yourself that moving the body helps level out hormones and regulate stress, so incorporating a routine exercise program into your day is essentially planting the seeds for a physically and mentally empowering, calm, and gorgeous pregnancy. I cannot stress enough that a healthy body yields a healthy mind.

baby on the brain

When I found out I was pregnant I was absolutely elated. I couldn't believe that something I had dreamed about for so many years was finally coming true. But mixed with the elation were flashes of anxiety. What if I'm not a good mom? What if something is wrong with the baby? Should I breast-feed or bottle-feed? How will I handle my career and a child? My reality was a whirlwind of uncertainty; nothing seemed to have a floor beneath it. It was a surreal situation, but I quickly realized that I had no choice but to surrender to the state of unknowing. And it was not easy to surrender when my hormones had me on an emotional roller coaster. I was up. I was down. I laughed. I cried. Now, I'm sure I'm

EATING FOR ENERGY

I'll say it again: Finding the energy to exercise is going to be a challenge during this trimester. But if you take the time to fuel yourself properly, you'll gain more pep in your step. Try these quick and easy ways to energize yourself through food:

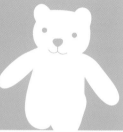

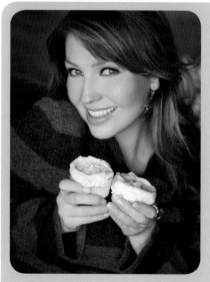

✳ A well-balanced breakfast daily is key, such as a warm bowl of oatmeal with calcium-fortified low-fat milk (or soy milk), berries, and almonds; or egg whites scrambled with chives and low-fat cream cheese.

✳ If you're short on time (who isn't?), blend up a smoothie of fruit, yogurt, and honey; you can even toss in your prenatal supplements or any other vitamins you may be taking.

✳ Drink plenty of fluids. Since hydration equals energy, aim to drink at least eight glasses a day in the form of juice, water, or clear broth. If this is a challenge for you, suck on ice cubes, or make ice cubes from your favorite juices.

✳ Eat most of your meals during the day; eat less at night.

✳ Although we want to keep sugars in check, every once in a while it's nice to treat your-self to something you love (in moderation, of course). Have that scoop of ice cream, nibble on that muffin top, or lick the frosting off a cupcake if that's what makes you happy. Don't think that you must deprive yourself entirely.

not the only new mom to grapple with these emotions, anxieties, and questions. But when I was in the midst of these turbulent feelings, I felt so alone. Luckily I discovered some powerful tools to help me overcome the hardest moments.

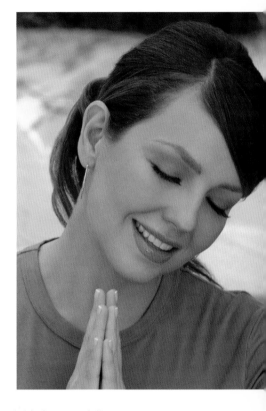

As I did during my first trimester, you may be feeling isolated or anxious. You may be worried about the baby's health (or your own). You may want to throw your partner off a balcony for saying the wrong thing. Or maybe you're still in total shock over the fact that you are going to be someone's mother, knowing that you can barely keep your aloe plant alive. Pregnancy is replete with highs, lows, and everything in between. But you can take charge and change your state of mind from sullen gray skies to a flood of sunshine. If you know what to expect psychologically, you are likely to find solace and solutions much faster.

You have to be solution-oriented when you're pregnant, and this is especially true when it comes to matters of the mind. Sometimes the simplest things can help, like listening to music that makes you happy if you're feeling down. Play reggae, Mozart, '80s music, salsa, whatever gets your dance face on. If you suddenly feel anxious, take five really long, slow breaths with your eyes closed, or take a soothing shower. If you feel isolated, tell your partner to hold you and pamper you a bit, and make that part of the prenatal regimen. If you start to experience identity issues, try keeping a journal or make lists of all your values and the positive things in your life. Try starting each page of the journal with a positive affirmation about yourself and your love for the baby.

If you fear the unknown, as many women do, practice trusting the universe and know that everything is unfolding exactly as it should. Be open, be flexible, and be accepting.

Many women also fear having a miscarriage, which is totally natural. The best thing you can do is reframe the sentiment by thinking positively about your baby. Keep telling yourself that you are a strong and sturdy home for your baby.

Some pregnant women experience relationship issues, as couple dynamics start to shift with a baby on the way. Keeping the romance alive with sexy dates is always a good idea, and ask your partner to speak to you softly, gently. Commit to keeping an open line of communication at all times. If you don't feel sexy, remember that sexy is on the inside. You know how to make your lover happy. You can show him he's not getting lost in the pregnancy shuffle.

If you feel shock, regret or an overwhelming sense of excitement, deep breaths are in order again, as well as acceptance that your life is beautiful and the life within you is nothing short of divine. Pregnant women endure all varieties of emotional turbulence, but fighting the dark side with positive actions and thoughts definitely makes the ride smoother.

What I found most fascinating (and confusing) about pregnancy is that it is such a paradox. At one moment you might feel empowered by the fact that you are strong enough to carry a child, yet incredibly vulnerable because of all the possible dangers that can affect a growing fetus. You might feel hopelessly depressed because all you want to do is sleep, but then again grateful that sleep brings sweet relief. You may find yourself at odds with your partner for any number of reasons one morning, and that very night feel closer to him than ever.

All of your feelings are valid, and the key to emotional survival during this wild period is to recognize that each feeling of dread and every moment of angst will eventually pass.

My mantra in times of distress was "I'm under the influence of my hormones." When you keep this at the forefront of your mind, you will suffer far less. Easier said than done, you might be thinking to yourself. So spend time practicing stress-reducing activities—that will make time pass more quickly and you will feel even better.

In this emotional tornado, you can help yourself more than anyone else can. I highly recommend finding a stress-relieving practice that's right for you. If you are the cynical type who scoffs at yoga or meditation, I encourage you to open your mind. But these practices are not the only things that work. During these nine months, you should feel free to get creative about how you relax, and whatever techniques you choose can help to restore your peace of mind and bring you back to mother-to-be-bliss.

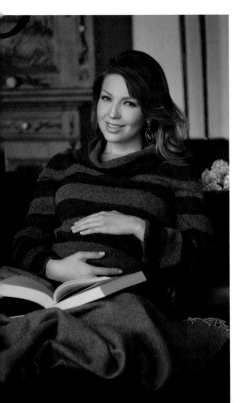

express yourself

Keeping a journal is a creative and therapeutic way to process your feelings and anxieties. It is also a nice way to zero in on how your mood changes day to day, especially if you designate the same time each day to write, such as first thing in the morning, when you are ripe with all of the night's dreams, fears, emotions, and anxieties. Drain the brain by writing everything down. Take it one step further by attaching all of your sonograms, doctor's notes, and pre-scriptions, making your journal more of a multidimensional scrapbook. You will be surprised at how much lighter you will feel when you release a lot of that frantic energy in the form of words on paper, and, even better, you will have your own personal archive of your pregnancy.

go inside

If the word "meditation" intimidates you, freaks you out, or puts you off, call it something else and give it a whirl anyway. There is nothing more soothing than some conscientious quiet time to calm the nerves and deeply reflect. And your first trimester is an ideal time to undo the shackles of the everyday and spend some time with just yourself (and your baby, of course).

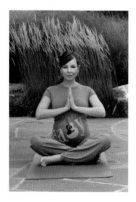 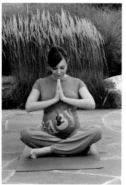 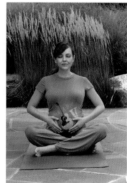 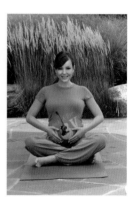

A simple and effective way to approach meditation, especially for first-timers, is to sit quietly with your eyes closed and simply observe your breath as it moves into your nasal passage, into your upper chest, and all the way down into the pit of your stomach. Observe every detail of your breath: Is it cold? Does it move freely? Is it going into one nostril or both? Monitor your breath as if it were the only thing in the world. Just by staying aware of your breath, and nothing else, you will notice how your mind will naturally start to quiet and your nerves begin to calm. The key to proper breath awareness is to observe the exact moment of "the switch" from inhale to exhale. That little tiny space can be a tremendous tool for a deep meditation. The next step is to scan your body for any sensations—be they cold, sweaty, tingly, numb, tender, sore—and instead of reacting to sensations, simply let them come and go. Some will surely linger longer than others, but eventually they all pass. Think of your problems as clouds wafting by, or try this: Imagine that your mind is a crystalline river and that you are placing your problems in a straw basket to lower into the river. Let the running water cleanse the basket of its emotional debris.

If you can train yourself to do this once a day, for at least fifteen to twenty minutes, you will develop a deep sense of awareness. Gradually, you will build a sense of conscious tranquility that will benefit you far beyond the birth of your baby.

baby bonding

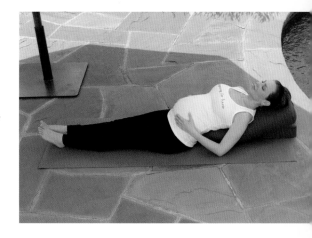

Simply lie down in total stillness with your palms on your belly. Make the setting comfy: Use a pillow under your knees for lower-back support, light scented candles, and play meditative music. (Some of my favorites are Colin Willsher's *Zen Garden: The Art of Wellbeing*, Raya Yoga's *Music for Positive Thinking*, and Michael Jones's *The Living Music*.) Though you may not feel your baby moving during the first trimester, by bringing your awareness to him, you are already bonding with him. I would put both of my hands on my belly and just lie there listening to my heartbeat, which I knew I was sharing with my child, even though she was the size of a thimble. I would look forward to this quiet personal time with my baby and take comfort in these sessions, essentially our first dialogues with one another.

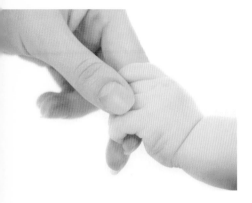

see to believe

Visualization exercises can be very useful as a grounding tool. Start with the breathing exercises described previously, and then allow yourself to start seeing in your mind's eye what your baby looks like inside of you. When you attempt to envision your baby growing, from a little seed to the shape of a tiny bouncing bean, to having little arms and eyes, to having a head—you get further away from your own preoccupations and closer to the true appreciation of the miracle of life and your role in it. I did these visualizations to the point where I could scan my baby's entire body, all her little parts, itemizing them one by one, and even go inside and see her precious healthy organs—heart, lungs, bones. I would wrap her in a bubble of light and love and keep that image close to my heart.

move what your mama gave ya

Prenatal yoga is a fantastic way to keep moving and stretching throughout pregnancy (see "Prenatal Yoga," page 50); but if you can't make it to a yoga class every day, do some figure 8s with your hips as often as you can. It keeps the joints loose and the hips open. I did them every day—in the shower, while waiting in line, in elevators. (Now that the baby is a few months old, I still do those figure 8s with her in my arms, and it puts her right to sleep.)

sing it, sister

For me, singing is therapy. You might think it's crazy, but I got myself a karaoke machine and sang my pregnant heart out when I felt anxious. Everything from Céline Dion to Gloria Estefan. It calmed me and invigorated me all at once. Consider it yoga for your soul.

beauty is in the eye of the baby holder

You know how people always say pregnant women look radiant? Well, during my first trimester I felt anything *but* radiant. My skin was spotty, my eyes looked tired, and I felt bloated and uncomfortable. But I couldn't hide inside for twelve weeks. So, using all the tricks I've learned through the years from stylists and makeup artists around the world, I pulled myself together and got out the door. And you know what? Looking good actually made me feel good. In this section I share with you some of my favorite tips for putting your best self forward during the challenging first trimester.

Remember that taking care of yourself does not end at diet and exercise; in fact, pampering, adorning, indulging, and beautifying yourself are all key acts of what I like to call self-glorification, a state of mind that invites you to take every opportunity to celebrate your beauty. Tap into your goddess and let yourself dabble freely with makeup, accessories, hairstyles, and fashion.

the skin you're in

If you are one of the lucky ones, you might find that you've never loved your skin more than when you are pregnant. Because the body is pumping more blood as it works to create life, for some women the result is a radiant, rosy complexion. The pregnancy glow (which, for nine whole months, is totally *free*) is the number one tool to work with as you strive for style.

But like many women, you may also experience heightened skin sensitivity and skin changes, such as oiliness or discoloration. Below the neck, you may even start to notice dark lines between the pubic bone and navel, and bursts of tiny spider veins in the legs. The best thing you can do to deal with these conditions is to accept the fact that they all usually fade after pregnancy. The stretch marks don't entirely disappear, but that's life. Think of them as the mother of all battle scars and yourself as the ultimate she-warrior.

No matter what changes your skin undergoes, remember that there are things you can do to enhance its appearance. The first rule, of course, is that true luminosity radiates from within, so *feeling* good will fuel your glow more than any lotion, cream, gel, or mask. That, however, does not mean you should not be fully pampering the largest organ of your entire body—your skin.

✳ **Lizard queen:** If you have patches of dry skin, let yourself splurge on a moisturizer that you adore. Use it twice daily, and double the amount of water you are drinking.

✳ **Grease monkey:** If you are oily, try carrying sheets of those powdery, oil-absorbing papers to blot the face. Available in packs, they're portable, easy, and a lifesaver when you're on the go. You may not find them at your local drug store, but specialty beauty stores like Sephora will definitely carry them.

✳ **X marks the spot:** One of the less pleasant things in life is adult acne. And the condition is all the more awful when you feel tubby to begin with. Fat and zit-laden is no one's favorite combo. To tame these tiny face monsters in a safe and natural way, avoid consuming oils and using oily face products. Wash your face throughout the day to keep the skin clean and fresh. For large blemishes, slice a washed grape in half and rub it right on the blemish; this is a fantastic, aromatic, and natural remedy for stubborn pimples. Stay far away from the acne treatments Retin-A, Tetracycline, and especially Accutane, which is known to cause birth defects.

✳ **Itching for relief:** Many women report extreme skin itchiness when they are pregnant, which is easily quelled by soaking in a warm oatmeal bath and by wearing breathable cotton clothes. You can also try to quell the itchiness with hydrocortisone creams in varying strengths, depending on how bad the itch is.

❋ **The stretch mark story:** In my line of work, stretch marks are just not an option, and I knew I would have to do everything in my power to prevent them. Thankfully, I found a fabulous cream called La Roche-Posay Active C Emulsion Light, which has helped to combat stretch marks. I recommend trying many different creams and seeing what works best for you.

THE SAY-GOOD-BYE-FOR-NOW LIST

Pampering your skin is great, but being mindful of your pregnancy is better—and far more important. There are some products and cosmetic treatments that you might want to hold off on until a month or so after you deliver. While we don't know for certain if these things are harmful for expectant mothers or developing fetuses, it is best to err on the side of caution. Vanity shmanity, your baby comes first.

Avoid the following treatments and products:

❋ Acrylic nails

❋ Botox

❋ Glycolics or peelings

❋ Herbal body wraps

❋ Laser removal of pubic hair

❋ Sunless self-tanners

the mane idea

Many women find that part of "the glow" includes a new and unexpected head of thicker, richer, more luxuriant hair. Work that fresh new mane by treating yourself to more salon visits and maybe even experimenting with new styles. I did the whole pregnancy thing by the book, so there were no highlights for me. But you can still get dynamic: If you've worn it short for the last eight years, this might be a nice time to let it grow out;

conversely, if you've always had long hair, a shorter style might freshen you up and add a sense of lightness and pep to your step.

There are all kinds of arguments and no real conclusive studies about certain hair treatments, such as perms, relaxers, and dyes, and their link to birth defects. Many believe the chemicals used in some of these products are so strong that, when left on the scalp for too long, they can move into the bloodstream and affect the developing fetus. Maybe I'm just old-fashioned when it comes to this stuff, but I like to err on the side of prudence when it comes to *anything* that includes the words "risk" and "birth defects" in the same breath. If you are dying for a dye job, buck up and at least wait until your first trimester is over, since it really is the most critical stage for the development of the fetus. Also, check in with your doctor about any treatment you are considering having at any time during your term.

breast friends

Mark my words: Your boobs will be two of your favorite things about being pregnant. Flat girls all of a sudden will have luscious handfuls, and the cups of voluptuous women will overfloweth like never before. While you are pregnant, your breasts will enter a whole new dimension. Not only will they be larger, but your nipples may also darken and you may experience breast sensitivity. This happens because of the increased hormonal activity in the body and blood flow to the breasts specifically. Breast sensitivity is one of the most common symptoms of pregnancy and also something that typically happens early on, given the hormonal flux and increased blood flow to the bosom.

There's nothing sexier than a hint of cleavage peeking from your blouse. So while you've got it, I say flaunt it! You'll probably need a new bra in a bigger size. So head to your favorite lingerie store; a sexy little number can go a long way in making you feel like a hot mama. Later on, practical but sexy nursing bras will be the most helpful. I won't lie to you: For the second, third, and fourth trimesters you will need industrial-strength support, but in the interim, enjoy the sensuality and see your breasts as the supreme signposts of glorious womanhood.

Other, subtler (and less pretty) changes may occur during this first trimester. Your belly might not be as flat or as tight as it normally is, you might feel a bit on the bloated side, and you might have a bit more to grab on to in the hips and buttocks. Savor the fact that you at least still have a waist to belt in these early weeks, and strut your (quickly evolving) curves with pride.

is she or isn't she?

Because there is so much going on inside of you in the first trimester, it's nice to really celebrate outwardly by looking great. And since you essentially still have your figure, you can reap the perks of pregnancy (the "glow," the hair, the breasts) and still appear to not be pregnant at all—which works fabulously for women who, for whatever reasons, want to conceal their pregnancies for as long as possible. I know I did. In fact, I waited almost five months before I told anyone outside of my immediate family, perhaps as my own personal way of honoring whatever was to come and having profound respect for the delicate process. I wanted the pregnancy to be my private pact with Creation itself, until I was ready to begin sharing and celebrating the news.

But until then, I found some cheeky ways to keep my cover . . .

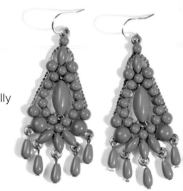

✳ **Optical illusions:** In the first few weeks of my pregnancy I became a master illusionist, drawing as much attention as possible to my face and hair, thereby distracting from my bump. I let myself go totally glam with eye makeup and always made sure my lips were freshly glossed; I went for big, sexy hair and long, dangly earrings. I wore off-the-shoulder tops that featured my neck. By keeping the action upstairs, I simply didn't give anyone a reason to look down.

✳ **Liven up:** In general, the more active you are, the less likely people are to wonder, "What's going on with you?" So inasmuch as you can handle it, stay busy, active, and social, always making sure to get enough rest and relaxation, but also staying on the ball with your friends and family. If you don't exactly feel like the Energizer Bunny, it's perfectly fine to tell people you are feeling under the weather during the first few weeks.

✳ **White lies:** Before you leave the house, think of what you are going to say to people when they ask why you aren't having a drink. "I have an early morning meeting" or "I am on a diet and counting calories" or "I'm taking a yoga class at seven AM" are all viable answers. Decide what your story is going to be for the night, and stick with it. Remember, it's nobody's business but your own.

pregnancy chic

The first rule of Pregnancy Chic is to abandon all your preconceived notions of what looks good on you. Pre-pregnancy, you may never have been the kind of gal to wear clingy clothes, but as you ease into your quickly morphing shape, you will come to

MEMO TO THE WORLD VS. MUM'S THE WORD

There are women out there whose cell phones do not have enough battery life to endure the manic flurry of phone calls they will want to make the moment they find out that they are going to have a baby. These women will have the news on the tip of their tongue, eager to share it with anyone who will listen. They will wear their pregnancy loud and proud, delighted by their achievement, joyful for the journey. Other women, however, might not be so keen on spilling the beans, wanting to keep the news under wraps for a bit longer before making the big announcement. Some women will wait three months, others will wait three minutes, and ultimately, both stances are totally valid.

When to tell people about your new addition is entirely personal. It is your body, your baby, and your choice as to when you decide to break the news. In many ways I could not wait to share it, and yet I forced myself to wait a full five months before I made my pregnancy public. But I had my reasons: The world that I work in can be brutal media-wise, so I figured it would be most sensible to keep the pregnancy as low-profile as possible. I wanted to be safe and get way past the initial, most delicate phase of the pregnancy, just in case anything happened.

On the other hand, many women want a full entourage of support in place from the get-go and might feel the need to start telling people right away. The common practice is to wait out the first three months, getting past the stage when miscarriage is the greatest risk. No matter what you decide, after a certain amount of time you won't be able to hide it, whether you want to or not.

realize that body-hugging silhouettes are now more flattering than that baby-doll dress. I found it ironically delightful that the curvier I got, the better I seemed to look in my sexiest outfits, as if I were always meant to be this voluptuous, a full expression of my womanhood at last. I realized that big can be beautiful, especially if one knows some of the tricks of the trade.

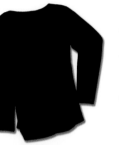

Pregnancy style is equal parts confidence, personal aesthetics, and willingness to try new ideas. But keeping your finger on the pulse of fashion while you shape-shift isn't always easy, so here are a few basic suggestions for what I think are perennial fashion essentials for the first trimester:

bump-wear 101

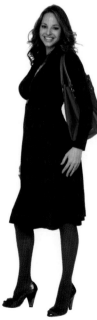

✳ **Working girl:** At the office, boyish looks like sharp tailored suits or crisp white button-down shirts are fantastic to keep your wardrobe polished and fresh. They play nicely against the feminine shape of the pregnant frame and help cover up an early pregnancy. Structured jackets and blazers are also great for hiding the early bump and giving contour to the body.

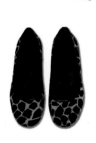

✳ **Lounging lady:** Leggings rule because they are perfect with dresses, tunics, and boots. Long cotton dresses are also ideal for concealing the not-quite-a-bump-yet belly and also for elongating the body. Easy separates like comfortable T-shirts and long tank tops are great. Remember that first-trimester clothes will also likely be useful in your fourth trimester—so think of them as a transitional wardrobe.

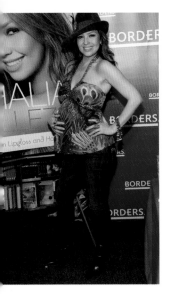

✳ **Pregn-elegant:** Form-fitting shapes that reveal curves are sexy, whereas baggy clothes create a stockier frame. So start to look for clothing that will hug your body. Dramatic earrings draw attention to your face and away from your belly. Accessories, too, are a great way of diverting attention from an unfamiliar outfit choice by keeping the focus on the funky accents, whether a leopard-print purse, a slick fedora, or those drop chandelier earrings that make you feel like a star.

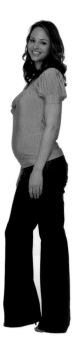

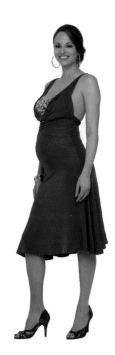

Every day, before you get dressed, remind yourself that:

✳ Pregnant does not equal boring.

✳ The glow is gorgeous.

✳ My beauty comes from inside me.

✳ I can still turn heads.

getting ready

We already know that the first three months are all about big changes. We've talked quite a bit about the body and mind. But what about the prospect of *getting ready for a baby*? Well . . . start thinking in baby steps, and gracefully acknowledge that for the next forty weeks, you will find yourself making a long list of important choices. Even though the birth day is a good six or more months away, now is the time to take the necessary prenatal tests, start thinking about who you want on your medical team, and decide when you will tell your friends and family the good news.

timeframe: nuts and bolts

The forty-week pregnancy timetable begins on the first day of your last menstrual cycle. A normal full-term pregnancy is from thirty-seven weeks to forty-one weeks. After forty-one weeks a pregnancy is considered a post-dates pregnancy and complication rates increase. Therefore, additional testing might need to be done to assure the well-being of the fetus. A normal, full-term pregnancy can vary. Babies are usually born within two weeks of the estimated due date.

While you may not notice any outward changes during the first trimester, which encom-passes the first thirteen weeks (or the first three months), this period is critical in the development of the embryo and later the fetus. By the sixth or seventh week an ultrasound can usually detect your baby's heartbeat, and by the eighth week, the placenta forms and begins to function. During this time your baby develops tiny webbed fingers and toes. The first trimester is considered the most crucial period of development. But it's also the riskiest for birth defects, so, for this reason, it is critical to be armed with all of the right information up front.

prenatal screening and testing

On the purely scientific end of the spectrum, the first trimester is the time for some critical analysis, known as prenatal testing. There are several tests, some of them necessary and some optional. This section will give you a rough idea of what the tests are, the reasons they're important, and the timeline for taking them. Having your team in place will make it easier to sift through and make sense of all the options. Although you and your partner will ultimately be the ones to make the call, an informed healthcare provider like your ob-gyn (and the input of your midwife, if you have one) should be your chief source of counsel regarding which tests are appropriate for you. It's too difficult, and totally unnecessary, for you to make these choices on your own.

facing complications

Though this is the section that no one wants to talk about, it is important—for both your physical and your mental health—to stay informed about the types of complications that can arise. While many of them might be scary to even consider, having the right information will help prepare you to deal with them if they do come up. Let's start with some of the basics:

✳ **Anemia:** An iron deficiency, anemia is quite common and also very manageable. It won't necessarily harm the baby, though some studies have associated anemia with low birth weight or preterm labor. Feeling consistently exhausted is one sign of anemia. Be sure to tell your doctor if you're experiencing this symptom; he or she will likely instruct you to eat more iron-rich foods, such as red meat, oatmeal, and dark leafy greens, or to take a daily iron supplement.

✳ **Ectopic pregnancy:** We know that the fertilized egg needs to be implanted in the uterus for it to develop properly, but in 1 percent or less of all pregnancies the egg will attach itself elsewhere, usually in the fallopian tube. This is a condition known as an ectopic pregnancy, that can be detected by seeing your gynocolgist early on and having an ultrasound five to seven weeks after your last period. Symptoms of an unruptured ectopic pregnancy include: vaginal bleeding or spotting along with abdominal pain (but don't panic because these symptoms can also occur with a healthy pregnancy). See your doctor early and have an ultrasound. However, if you also develop severe abdominal pain, shoulder pain, weakness, lightheadedness, dizziness, low blood pressure or a weak or erratic pulse you need to seek immediate medical attention. This is a life-threatening situation for the mother where the developing embryo has caused a rupture of the fallopian tube and the mother is now actively bleeding internally.

✳ **Fibroids:** Some women, especially those over age thirty-five, are at risk for fibroids, which are benign uterine growths usually seen during the first ultrasound. They are quite common among women with a family history and also among African American women. Depending on their size and location, fibroids are generally not harmful to pregnancies if they are located within the wall of the uterus or attached and grow outward from the surface of the uterus. In some cases, fibroids can grow quite rapidly during pregnancy and cause great discomfort or pain due to a process known as degeneration, and could require hospitalization and narcotic pain relief. Fibroids that are located within the uterine cavity can cause even more serious problems, and women with this type of fibroid, known as a sub-mucous fibroid, are usually advised not to get pregnant until it/they are removed. If a woman conceives with this type of fibroid it can increase the risk of miscarriage, breech births, preterm labor, or placenta previa—all of which can increase the chance of a C-section being needed. In addition, fibroids increase the risk for a C-section because these tumors can sometimes cause obstruction in the passageway. In other words, they can prevent the baby from descending the birth canal if they are large enough and located in the lowermost portions of the uterus and cervix. If you have fibroids, your healthcare provider will examine them for size and placement, then assess what course of action to take.

✳ **Gestational diabetes:** Another complication that can usually be treated by diet and exercise is gestational diabetes (also known as pregnancy induced diabetes), which is typically screened for at twenty-four to twenty-eight weeks (see "Basic Screening Tests," page 74). If you have a preexisting case of diabetes, it is extremely important that you work with a doctor who is specialized in that condition and who can assist you during your term and beyond. It is equally important that women with gestational diabetes see a dietician as well, as these women in particular may not be familiar with a diabetic diet and may need counseling on what foods they can and cannot eat to keep their blood sugars in a normal range. Whether you enter your pregnancy with a preexisting case of diabetes, or if you develop gestational diabetes, a dietician can assist you with the proper diet during your pregnancy.

basic screening tests

Generally, prenatal screening tests evaluate potential genetic, chromosomal, or other health issues, and they can determine gestational age, sex, and other basic information. Blood tests are typically done between weeks 9 and 11 to screen for hepatitis B, sexually transmitted diseases (STDs), antibodies, and cystic fibrosis and to check the mother's blood type. Ultrasounds are usually performed between weeks 11 and 13, using sound waves to create a picture of the developing fetus. Ultrasounds during the first trimester have several functions: They examine your reproductive organs, such as the ovaries, cervix, and uterus; determine the due date; determine the number of babies you're carrying; check the baby's heartbeat; and ensure that the baby is developing properly inside your uterus. When I first saw that bouncing little bean on the ultrasound monitor, I realized that I had not been hallucinating, that I would in fact be someone's mother. When I heard that life-affirming heartbeat, something inside me shifted, and I was never the same again.

The first-trimester ultrasound includes the nuchal translucency screening, which tests for Down syndrome by looking for an increased space in the back of the neck, which can indicate chromosomal abnormalities. If that measurement is high, women are often advised to have a fetal echocardiogram (an ultrasound reading of the baby's heart) to check whether things are developing normally. Down syndrome is one of the more common birth defects, affecting one in one thousand babies, and becomes more likely as the mother's age increases.

Pap smears and urine cultures are also typically done as routine prenatal tests. None of these standard tests pose any risk to the baby, and the results can be useful in deciding whether to pursue additional diagnostic tests.

diagnostic tests

Women with high-risk pregnancies may be candidates for more diagnostic tests. If an abnormality (such as an increased nuchal thickness) is detected during your first trimester ultrasound, you will most likely be offered a chorionic villus sampling (CVS), which is an early test that allows you to know sooner rather than later whether your child is affected by a genetic abnormality such as Down syndrome or cystic fibrosis (see "More Prenatal Screening and Testing," page 88). However, because the CVS is done earlier in the pregnancy (at weeks 10–12), it allows you to know sooner rather than later if you are at risk for serious birth defects, which in some cases might even be a reason to terminate the pregnancy. The CVS entails taking a sample of cells from the placenta (through the vagina or the abdomen, depending on where the placenta is situated) and is typically performed in a hospital or in the offices of doctors trained in this procedure.

Though the test is almost 100 percent accurate, people are often wary of it, as it brings the slight risk of miscarriage (one in two hundred women). If you're faced with deciding on whether to do a CVS, consider your individual risk factors such as family history and age, and make the decision after speaking with your obstetrician and possibly even a genetic counselor. You should also take comfort in the fact that by waiting until after week 10, and by finding a reliable testing center with an excellent track record, you do increase your chances of a safe and effective CVS test.

the age-old question

I remember panicking when I learned that women have a finite number of eggs. I worried that maybe being in my thirties would negatively impact my pregnancy. Thankfully, medical advances have made the prospect of having a baby at a later age viable and safe for both the mother and the baby. And indeed, I ultimately gave birth to a healthy 9-pound baby at age thirty-six, feeling great and looking great. The key is to stay

FIRST-TRIMESTER TESTS

WHEN	WHY	RISK
Blood tests weeks 9–11	to screen for chromosomal abnormalities such as Down syndrome by measuring levels of hCG and the pregnancy-associated plasma protein A, known as PAPP-A	none
Ultrasound weeks 11–13	to check mother's uterus, cervix, and ovaries; the number of babies; the baby's heartbeat; and confirm that the pregnancy is in the proper location. It is important to have an early ultrasound to rule out an ectopic pregnancy (a pregnancy outside the uterus which can be a life threatening condition).	none
CVS weeks 10–13	to detect almost all of the disorders for which abnormal genes or chromosomes are responsible	1 in 200 women miscarry
NT ultrasound weeks 10–13	Weeks 10–13 screen for Down syndrome as well as other abnormalities. An increased NT increases the risk for Down syndrome, so if you present with this, you should consider having an amnio or CVS. An increased NT also increases the risk for heart defects so you should consider having a detailed sonogram of the baby's heart (called a fetal echo) at 20–22 weeks.	none
Combined screening weeks 10–13	to detect Down syndrome and other abnormalities with increased accuracy by combining maternal blood screening and NT ultrasound	none

informed and take all necessary precautions. If you or your baby present any serious conditions, healthcare providers will monitor the pregnancy more closely and advise you of all your options.

IF YOU'RE AN EXPECTANT MOTHER IN YOUR THIRTIES, TAKE PRIDE BECAUSE . . .

✳ You are already self-realized. You have accomplished many of your dreams by now.

✳ You are more mature than you could ever have been in your twenties.

✳ You are more confident and capable of dealing with pain and adversity.

✳ You are more informed about the ins and outs of pregnancy because you have seen it around you.

Genetic counseling is the way you will learn the most about potential problems early on in the pregnancy. These types of counselors are trained to assess the parents' genetic profiles and to help expectant parents understand risks that may lie ahead given family history, screening results, and other variables, like maternal age or exposure to certain medications, toxins, or radiation. Genetic counseling, during which parents-to-be can determine their odds of having a healthy baby, is typically encouraged if there is a better-than-average chance that both parents carry the gene for a specific disorder or if someone in the family (brother, sister, cousin) has any genetic or developmental (anatomical) abnormality. Some of these disorders are linked to geography and ethnicity, such as Tay-Sachs in Eastern European Jews, or sickle-cell anemia in African Americans. Discuss your own scenario with your healthcare provider first so that together you can assess whether this type of counseling is appropriate for you. If it is, your doctor can refer you to a specialist.

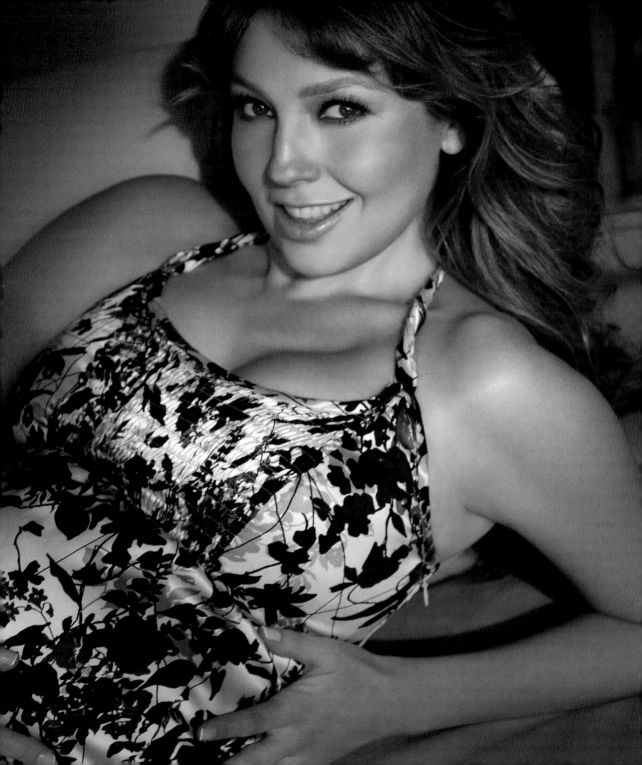

chapter 2: power mama rising

SECOND TRIMESTER: WEEKS 14–27/MONTHS 4–6

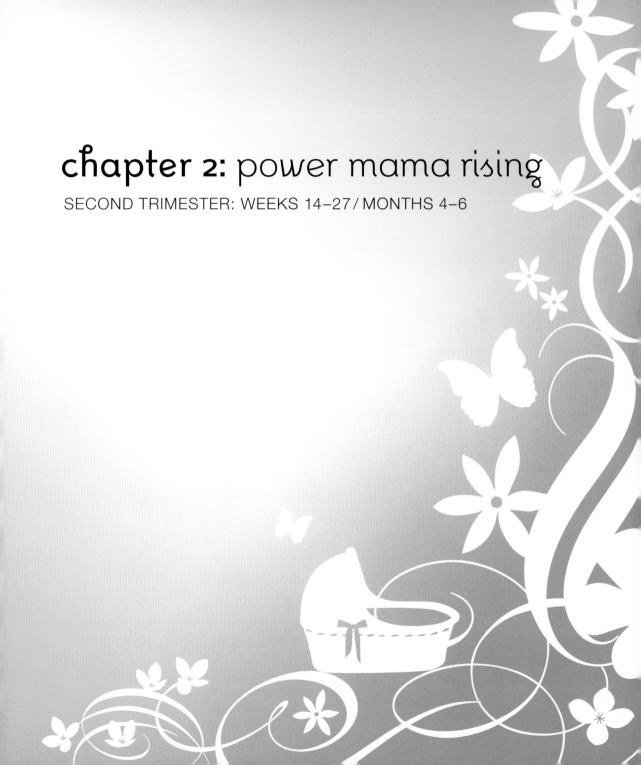

After the pukes and exhaustion of the first trimester

of pregnancy, the second trimester is simply fantastic. For me it felt like a perfect place in my life. I had confidence, renewed energy, and unstoppable hope. I was proud that I had made it through the challenges of the first few months. After thirteen weeks of discomfort, nonstop vomiting, and total exhaustion, the second trimester felt like a glimmering light at the end of the tunnel—the first of many lights that would continue to shine for me. By week 14, I felt as though I had gotten to a point where I somehow knew *how* to be pregnant, where life with my baby became *normal*; by this time and beyond, my pregnancy started to feel absolutely delicious.

This chapter covers health issues and changes that occur as you progress into the term, how your baby is developing, what you should be eating (and not eating), what you might be thinking about, and what you *should* start thinking about as you enter the second trimester. We will also look at ways to feel fit and fabulous as your shape continues to shift.

This second trimester is full of so much—more joy, more energy, more fun, better appetite, better sleep, and yes, ladies, even better sex. But more important, it starts to put you in a strong, positive headspace—the very best place to be as you continue to prepare for your baby. With everything that you're juggling, the one thing that shines the brightest during your second trimester is the fact that motherhood is becoming more and more real. Your body is changing fast, your baby is growing rapidly, and the reality of it all is finally sinking into your mind.

keep building your dream team

Because things were relatively calm during this trimester, I was able to think about issues that I knew I would not have time or energy for in the third and fourth trimesters. One of the things I started thinking about was what sort of support I would need after the baby was born. Did I want a baby nurse or did I want to try to do it all on my own? At first I was adamant about not hiring any help, insisting to anyone who dared to tell me otherwise that "Millions of women have it done it before me. I want to raise my baby myself!!!" Once I had the baby, though, it became clear to me that help of any kind was something to embrace (especially with the pains that I describe in the fourth trimester), not run from, and in the end I found myself scrambling to find the right person for the job.

Take this time to think about what sort of help you'll need after the baby comes. Think about whether you'd like your mother or another close relative to stay with you to help out. Think about when you'll have to return to work and what sort of care you'll need for your baby. Remember that the person you choose will be more than just a hired hand; she will be the one to help you watch and nurture your little treasure. You want to take the hiring of such a person very seriously.

First, it will help to know what your options are and the differences between them. For example, a baby nurse is usually a registered nurse (RN) who has medical training and expertise with newborns and babies, whereas a nanny is more like a specialist in infant care, without the medical background. Some women might feel a baby nurse is overkill if they already have a good pediatrician, but since everyone's needs are different, it's nice to know there are options.

Use the time and mental energy of these few months to do some initial research. Talk to your close friends and family members and get referrals. Maybe start interviewing a few people. Have your list of questions carefully thought through, and know which items on your list are deal-breakers or nonnegotiable. Here are some questions you might consider when interviewing nannies or baby nurses:

❋ How many babies have you worked with?

❋ What are your strengths and what are your weaknesses with regard to baby care?

❋ What is your medical background, and do you have experience with infant-related medical emergencies?

❋ Would you be willing to stay overnight?

❋ Would you feel comfortable knowing there is a camera in the baby's room?

❋ Will you be willing to help me out with some basic housework, like light cleaning and cooking, if need be?

❋ Will you be willing to respect and honor my ideologies about certain parenting-related issues?

❋ Will you be able to help me with breastfeeding issues?

NANNYTUDE

Imagine you interview a series of nannies and finally decide on one. And she is basically living in your house and assisting you with your new baby, when all of a sudden, the first week in your house, out of nowhere you pick up on the fact that she is actually giving you the cold shoulder—what I call nannytude. The woman you thought you hired is a totally different woman when the sun goes down. No one ever prepares you for that. There you are, thinking, "This is the most sacred moment of my life, I don't even know how to bathe my child yet, the very least you can do is be nice to me."

You just don't know who is going to turn on you, so make sure your interviewing and screening process gives you enough time to really get a good sense of your prospects.

Keep in mind that the very best baby nurses, midwives, and doulas book quickly and way in advance. Take advantage of the calm now to look around and see who and what you like, because as you move into your third trimester, things become more and more of a beautiful chaos . . .

dealing with discomforts

By week 14, many women have a new pep in their step, feeling more energized, invigorated, and happier. This newfound spirit of optimism is likely due to the fact that the nausea and vomiting has subsided, if not entirely ended. You're peeing less like a racehorse and more like a human, and you're not starting each morning with your head in the toilet. You might still be feeling some fatigue, which is totally normal and just your body's way of coping with the hard work of growing a baby within. In the second trimester, you may start to experience some constipation and increased heartburn as your digestive organs rearrange themselves, making way for your ever-expanding uterus.

The second trimester will bring many new sensations and changes. Just know that for every uncomfortable new symptom, there is always something you can do to address it, even if it is as simple as taking three deep breaths.

tips

Listed here are some of the most common ailments of the second trimester. To help you through each one, I've given a few suggestions that certainly worked for me.

❋ **Abdomen aches or headaches:** Try lukewarm compresses on your forehead to relieve headaches, and try lying down to relieve the abdominal pain.

✳ **Anemia:** Take iron supplements, but be sure to ask your doctor about dosage. Too much iron can be harmful.

✳ **Bleeding gums (also known as "pregnancy gingivitis"):** When you're pregnant, your gums bleed due to fluctuating hormone levels, specifically higher progesterone levels, which make your gums more sensitive to the bacteria in plaque. Bleeding gums are also due to the increased blood supply to your mouth—and everywhere else in your body. To keep your gums healthy, floss daily and use a softer toothbrush. See your dentist, and get your teeth cleaned regularly.

✳ **Breast enlargement:** Get yourself an arsenal of new bras. Try to find styles that are at once sexy and supportive. This way you're addressing the issue but also having fun with your new endowments.

✳ **Constipation:** You may find that you're not as regular as you once were. The constipation is caused by digestive organs shifting to make room for the baby. Unpredictable bowel movements are the result. For this reason, it's essential to keep your digestive system in good working order. Drink prune juice, eat papaya, and take in plenty of brown rice, all of which are great sources of fiber. Other high-fiber foods include whole wheat bread, ground flax seeds, and kiwis. A pregnant woman needs 30 milligrams of fiber a day. Most important, drink at least 40 ounces of water daily.

✳ **Dizziness or faintness:** Go outside for fresh air, or sit down and close your eyes briefly until the sensation passes.

✳ **Faster pulse and shortness of breath:** It is normal to feel volatile and even jittery at times, since your heart is now beating faster and more forcefully. The sensation of being short of breath does not mean you are low on oxygen; it happens, instead, because the enlarging uterus has pushed many of the abdominal organs upward, so it takes greater effort to move your diaphragm downward against this increased resistance, making it seem like you are short of breath. Control your breathing by taking long, deep inhalations, counting to six for each inhale as well as for each exhale. Do sets of ten each morning and night.

✳ **Gassiness and bloating:** Continue to stay away from gassy foods (beans, broccoli, cauliflower) and sparkling beverages—and learn to live with it, because this symptom is going to be around for a while.

✳ **Hemorrhoids:** Constipation, or just the pressure in the pelvic region, can have any number of side effects, including hemorrhoids. Try cold compresses and witch hazel pads to relieve the burn, and take stool softeners (Colace is great) so you don't have to work so hard.

✳ **Nasal congestion and nosebleeds:** The increase in mucus production can lead to stuffiness. Up your vitamin C intake and plug a humidifier into your room.

✳ **Swelling feet, hands, and face:** No pregnancy goes without a certain amount of water retention. Wear comfortable shoes and drink fluids all day. Try to avoid foods and beverages that contain large amounts of sodium, such as chips or salted nuts, which causes water retention, and since you're skipping the sushi, you may as well strike the soy sauce, too.

✳ **Vaginal discharge:** Ignore it. This is just the result of increased vaginal secretions and cervical mucus production. Stay away from douches, as the chemicals they contain may be harmful.

✳ **Varicose veins:** Keep your feet elevated by putting a pillow under them when you can, for instance when you are in bed or relaxing on a couch. If they appear to be worsening, talk to your doctor about wearing compression stockings or panty-hose to prevent permanent damage to your veins.

By the fourth month (16 weeks), your baby is about 7 inches long and weighs about 5 ounces.

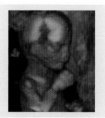

oh, baby!

You're not the only one who has come a long way by the second trimester—by the fourth month your baby is an entirely different creature. He is about 7 inches long, weighs about 5 ounces, has developed fingerprints and toe prints, and can put his finger in his mouth and even attempt to breathe. He has also developed temporary hair, which will fall off and change after birth. Later on in the trimester, by the fifth month, your fetus, weighing in at about a pound, has the ability to hear. He has facial features, including tiny eyebrows.

By the sixth month, the baby will be able to react to loud sounds and will open and close his eyes in reaction to light. (Yes, strong light can get through your body into the womb!) A protective coating called vernix caseosa will start to develop around his body. Your baby will also start to experience sleep-wake cycles, and his muscles and skeleton will continue to develop and strengthen. His body begins to move with more assertiveness, which you'll actually start to feel as kicks by the end of this trimester. Your fetus will grow to be 7 to 9 inches long—about half as big as it will be by the time he is born. If you are carrying a little boy, his testicles will have begun their descent from the abdomen into the scrotum.

more prenatal screening and testing

THE AMNIO For me, the word "amniocentesis" was a very scary word. When my doctor told me that this test entailed getting a long needle inserted into my pregnant belly, it sounded more like a cruel and unusual alien practice than a highly sensitive test. Dr. Kramer explained to me that the test would extract a sample of my amniotic fluid, which contains fetal cells, to evaluate the baby's deoxyribonucleic acid (DNA). Amniotic fluid is the colorless liquid that surrounds the baby in your uterus. It helps to protect and cushion your baby inside the amniotic sac. It also plays a vital role in the development of internal organs, such as the lungs and kidneys.

This test assesses the alpha-fetoprotein (AFP) and the main reason people opt for amniocentesis is to rule out genetic abnormalities such as Down syndrome or other genetic abnormalities if both mother and father are carriers for a specific genetic disease. Even though there is a one in two hundred chance of amniotic fluid leakage and a very slight risk of miscarriage, my doctor assured me that an amniocentesis is very safe and more than 99 percent accurate in ruling out some very serious problems.

Instead of freaking about the test, I started thinking of the word "amnio" as an abbreviation for "I am to know," helping to quell my fears—of birth defects, miscarriages, and needles. Though I struggled with whether I should have the test, and I did experience some mild cramping during the procedure itself, in the end I knew it was an important step in ensuring that I had a healthy pregnancy and baby.

Amniocentesis is optional and generally performed at around week 16, though some doctors perform it as early as week 15. You should consult your doctor to carefully analyze whether an amnio is right for you. You will need to consider many variables, including the results of your first-trimester screening tests, your age, and whether you had a CVS test, which also screens for chromosomal abnormalities like Down syndrome, as part of that first battery of tests. Some women have an amnio instead of a CVS because their ob-gyns have not been trained in CVS. Fewer ob-gyns can perform a CVS compared to an amnio, and if your ob-gyn does not do a CVS (and there is no one else in the region to whom they can refer you for this test) he or she will only offer an amnio.

Another benefit of the amnio was that, through chromosomal analysis, I could know with certainty the gender of my baby, as opposed to waiting for the week 20 ultrasound, which is not 100 percent accurate. My husband and I intuitively knew that we were going to have a girl, but having the amnio, dreadful as it seemed at first, gave us the stamp of certainty.

OTHER SECOND-TRIMESTER TESTS Because ultrasounds are noninvasive, many doctors also like to do a targeted, or Level 2, ultrasound at around weeks 18 to 22 as a routine evaluation to make sure your baby has developed properly. Today many women are also opting for 3-D ultrasounds, a technique that yields additional unique images of your baby. 3-D ultrasounds allow your doctors to see additional aspects of your baby's anatomy, which helps them rule out other problems. Just be aware that insurance companies often do not cover these, and they can cost upwards of $150.

Depending on which tests you received during your first trimester, your doctor may recommend a triple screen or quad screen, which look for several different things, such as Down syndrome and other chromosome problems. If these were ruled out by earlier screenings, your doctor will likely opt for just an AFP test to check for neural tube defects.

Between weeks 24 and 28, your doctor may offer you a standard glucose screening test, which looks for gestational diabetes (see page 73), a condition that occurs in 4 to 7 percent of pregnant women. The test determines whether a mother is producing enough insulin to process the extra glucose in her system. Gestational diabetes is highly treatable with diet modification and exercise.

positive head space

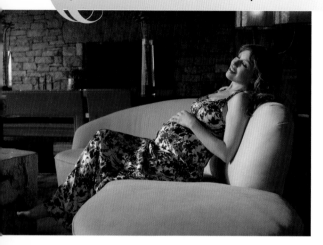

For me, the new feelings of joy and confidence that I began to experience in my second trimester further inspired me to *be good to myself*, so that I could quite naturally *be good to my baby*. Each day I made sure to take time for some sort of act of wellness, be it yoga, meditation, long walks, or even making love. I relished each day as if it were sacred, as if I were in my own private, prenatal spa, owned and operated by me, with myself as the sole, one and only, exclusive VIP member. It was a pampering like no other, but it was also a time of digging deep, spending lots of time with my mind, my body, my baby, and myself.

Trust me, I understand that it is a challenge to simultaneously juggle a career and a comprehensive wellness regimen; however, the latter is critical for the former to exist, and endlessly more important when you are pregnant. Do whatever you must to carve out even *fifteen minutes* each day for some personal time. I tried to start each day with visualizations, not only because I knew they were good for me, but also so that I could check that off my list right away. If I knew a busy day was ahead of me, I would try to set my alarm clock a half hour earlier to ensure that I would have time for the personal check-in each day that became my anchor throughout the term.

It is not uncommon to experience anxiety during these months, for any number of reasons: You might be too big, or not big enough; you may worry that the baby is not moving; you may start feeling anxious about what kind of parent you will be, or how you will co-parent with your partner; you might get all out of sorts over what kind of detergents to use on the baby's stuff, or what to feed the baby, or even how to calm the baby when she cries. You'll worry about it all. This is totally normal. First, remember that there is always a solution right around the corner, and by reading books like this one, cross-referencing information, and talking with your friends, family, and doctor and/or midwife, you will build the necessary foundation of guidance to keep you feeling properly informed.

When I found out with certainty that I was going to have a girl, everything changed . . . or everything started, I should say. My love affair with this little girl started that day, and from that moment on, I knew all of my decisions moving forward would ultimately be linked to her well-being. My husband also kicked into high gear. His nesting impulse all of a sudden became unstoppable; he cleaned, purged, edited, screened, dumped, and rearranged everything in sight, making way for *her*, our little princess who was on her way home.

Then again, you might find yourself feeling moody and even irritable instead of blissful and aglow. You may experience forgetfulness or find that you have trouble focusing. You might even feel anxious because you're not quite large enough to look exactly pregnant but feel oversize nonetheless. The good news is that there are ways to address all these feelings, which, as we know, in the end pass away.

visualization: let it play

If you're feeling out of sorts and scattered, a simple way to strengthen your focus and ground yourself is to spend time with visualization exercises. These exercises served as mental and emotional jet fuel as I prepared to give birth. I found that if I did them at the same time each day, the exercises became a stimulating routine, organically reset-ting my internal barometers of hope, confidence, awareness, and joy.

Here's what I visualized: I would close my eyes and, with my mind's eye, watch the scenes of my delivery unfold. I would visualize each step happening in perfect synchro-nicity, each beat, each moment a step toward the creation of what would ultimately become the beginning of *my family*. I would picture myself on the delivery table, my partner holding my hand, smiling at me; I would envision the flurry of nurses all hustling around me, cool and calm, quick and clean; I would think of my face all sweaty and even of how the screams would sound coming out of my mouth as I pushed. I would allow myself to imagine all of it, even little glimpses of the bits that terrified me, slowly, gently preparing myself for the event.

During this visualization, I would also talk to God to express gratitude. I would thank God for giving me the power to see and smell and touch and feel and ask Him to please do the same for my baby, and then I would envision the baby, healthy and happy, in my arms. I would think of all the women who are waiting to have babies, or those who are having trouble conceiving, or those waiting for adoption papers to come through, and I would feel the tremendous surge of gratitude. This visualization exercise gave me strength, helping me to quiet my mind, calm my breath, connect with my baby, and be with myself.

Whenever I was at a loss for which kind of visualization to do, I would refer to Gurmukh Kaur Khalsa's book (see "Resources," page 198), which has no shortage of ideas, insights, and inspiration.

DREAMING PREGNANT

If you think your waking life is intense when pregnant, your dream life can get even more intense. Not only does the flux of hormones affect your mind, but your own anxieties about motherhood are also harbored in your unconscious, where they can play themselves out however they please in your dreams.

I remember dreaming that my baby was part fish, some kind of mer-child. I had no idea what to make of it, but I was fascinated by it nevertheless. A friend of mine dreamed that her baby was born a cat. Some women dream about people from their past—former lovers or exes—which I understand as the unconscious mind working to clean its slate, making room for a new chapter. I like to think of dreams as magical flags: They signal something to our minds and spirits about what we need. Staying attuned to them is a great way to tap into our deepest self at a time when we need to the most. Writing down dreams is a great way to get the mind to remember them more consistently.

hydrotherapy: start fresh

In times of frustration or discomfort, I found hydrotherapy a big help in relieving negative feelings. One day I ran to the pharmacy and bought a bathing chair—the kind for geriatrics—parked my pregnant self in that chair, and let the shower water rain down on me for hours. The effects were calming, cleansing, and pretty much immediate.

The moment I would get an inkling of one of those negative or stress-causing thoughts sneaking in, I would get up and immediately take a shower or bath. To me, the act of washing has always been a way to let go of any negativity—maybe because by cleansing my body I'm symbolically cleansing my mind, or maybe because it just feels so good to do it. Water somehow relieves pain and fatigue, and at once calms and restores. There is nothing more rejuvenating than drawing a bath and soaking in it as the sounds of beautiful music swirl in the air with the aroma of lavender.

Of course, each woman should consult her doctor about water-temperature levels, but, generally speaking, by the second trimester your pregnancy is in a nice and sturdy place, making it easier for you to sit back in that tub, crank up your favorite soothing music, and really relax.

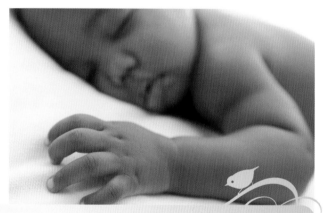

table for two: what to eat in the second trimester

By now, you have become a pro at taking your supplements, so this is the time to focus even more on making sure you eat the right foods in the right amounts and combinations to keep you and your baby nourished properly. For me, the second trimester was an opportunity to start anew, because during my first three months, I could barely keep anything down. But by the fourth month, my cravings and appetite kicked in, and

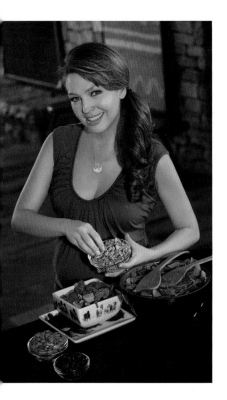

I decided to use that as an opportunity to pack in the right kinds of nutrients and the right amount of calories. Because each woman has a different frame and metabolism, try to determine with your doctor what your ideal pregnancy weight should be for each trimester and how many calories daily you will need to maintain it.

Since you are likely to be feeling better in your second trimester, you will probably go out a lot more. At restaurants, choose healthy entrées or change up the small things: Try to order brown rice instead of white, since whole grains contain the much-needed vitamins E and B and are excellent sources of fiber. Opt for salads, since green leafy vegetables are the best sources of carotenoids, which are critical for fetal development. Restaurants will usually add grilled chicken or salmon to almost any salad, which is a great way to get a hit of protein in the meal.

mo' h$_2$o

It's easy to forget to stay hydrated, and drinking glass after glass of water can, frankly, get boring. But by creating innovative libations, I found it was much easier to keep my body and baby adequately hydrated. I drank organic juices (guava and papaya especially) with splashes of seltzer water and rekindled my childhood love of fresh homemade lemonade. I drank chicken and veggie broths, and God knows I drank plenty of ginger tea. I stayed away from canned sodas and learned to love young coconut water, which is loaded with potassium and electrolytes, and pretty much tastes like a vacation. I would snack on watermelon slices or dice up a cucumber, both loaded with water. I always carried full bottles of water in the car.

So, to minimize bloating, skin problems, dehydration, moodiness, and a dozen other ailments, remember: You should be drinking an 8-ounce glass of liquid at least eight times per day.

protein

I tried to eat three servings of protein daily to achieve the recommended 60 to 75 grams. After one too many egg-white omelets, I let myself explore more, experimenting with simple, protein-packed dishes like miso-marinated tofu slices with avocado on multigrain toast, or barbecued turkey burgers on whole wheat buns, or spaghetti squash with a spicy Bolognese sauce, or a bowl of good ol' homemade chili.

Getting creative about your protein intake motivates you to eat the key foods that contain amino acids, the essential building blocks of human tissue. Don't forget that your baby needs protein to develop properly, and try to make the protein element the core of each meal.

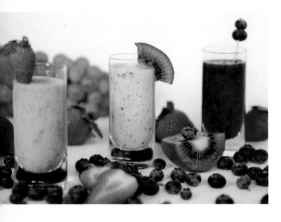

calcium

Make sure you also get four servings of high-calcium foods daily, which strengthens not only your baby's bones, but your own. Your baby is literally taking the calcium from your bones, so you have to replace it. I had a friend who thought this meant she should eat a pint of ice cream every night for six months—as you can imagine, this proved disastrous for her thighs. Her ever-expanding girth (and the aftereffects for many months beyond her delivery) taught me the invaluable lesson of knowing what kinds of calcium to consume.

Go for low-fat cheeses, milk, and yogurts or soy milk. Sesame seeds, almonds, and fortified orange juice are also excellent sources of calcium, as are broccoli, figs, and edamame.

GROOVY SMOOTHIE IDEAS by Esther Blum

BRAINIAC SMOOTHIE

1 cup frozen blueberries

1 cup plain Greek yogurt

1 tablespoon ground flax seeds

Blend together with ice. Will help fight momnesia (a.k.a. "baby brain").

THE MOVER AND SHAKER

1 cup plain almond milk

1 tablespoon natural peanut butter

1 cup strawberries or raspberries

2 tablespoons ground flax seeds

Cinnamon (to taste)

Blend together with ice. This shake boasts 10 grams of fiber and will help counteract the binding effects of the iron in the prenatal vitamins.

SATISFY-YOUR-CRAVING SMOOTHIE

1 cup milk, almond milk, or water

1 tablespoon almond butter or natural peanut butter

1 banana

1 tablespoon cocoa powder

1 tablespoon ground flax seeds

Blend together with ice and sprinkle additional cocoa powder on top. This shake will hopefully avert a binge on a pint of ice cream!

vitamin c

You also need to make sure you're getting plenty of vitamin C, which you'll find in all of the citrus fruits and many of the tropical fruits like guava, kiwi, papaya, mango, and pineapple. I became obsessed with making super-potent tropical smoothies that I could pack with fruit, adding protein powder and mixing in my prenatal vitamins. You can also get vitamin C from vegetables such as kale, arugula, asparagus, Brussels sprouts, and watercress.

Another really simple thing I would make for a vitamin C–packed, quick, nutritious, and cozy meal was to sauté an onion with a bit of garlic, then add a veggie such as chopped asparagus or broccoli, 2 cups of water, a chicken (or vegetarian) bouillon cube, and let that simmer five to eight minutes. Then I'd season it with a bit of salt and pepper and throw it in the blender for a fresh and delicious soup. I did this so many nights, with so many different vegetables, that there was always a fresh soup in my fridge that I could heat up in a mug for a meal or a snack. I can't lie: Soup and smoothies became my two best friends.

on the go and guilt-free

I'll say it again: If you don't have the time or energy to eat out or cook in, there are still many easy ways to eat healthy meals. Keep smart snacks in your purse and ensure that your cupboards are always stocked with:

* Air-popped popcorn

* Carrot-ginger soup

* Fresh, local fruits and veggies

* Hard-boiled eggs

* Lightly salted edamame

* Raw almonds, almond milk, and almond butter

* Ice cubes made of fruit juice

* Soy chips

* Soy nuts

* Sunflower and pumpkin seeds

* Whole grain cereals

* Whole wheat crackers

* Yogurt

power on

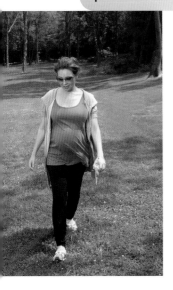

The second trimester is your opportunity to give it your all exercise-wise, because the first and third trimesters you are likely too sick and too big, respectively, to really work up a sweat. In your second trimester you can do the work that will make the weight and intensity of the third and fourth trimesters much less burdensome. With this in mind, fitness and exercise became a driving force for me, and I saw each workout as a step toward a stronger body and an easier delivery. I kept envisioning myself months after the birth, and I would see myself totally fit, lean, and limber. I knew that aside from my diet, consistent exercise would be my way of achieving this vision, so I used my newfound pep in the fourth month to really ramp up my fitness regimen.

The key to sticking to a program is to vary your exercise routine, keeping it active, dynamic, and daily. I made sure that my body was moving every which way every single day. Don't get me wrong, I rested plenty as well, but for at least forty-five minutes every day that I felt well enough, I would make it a point to find a way to move.

I also continued my prenatal yoga practice, which was enormously helpful to me both physically and mentally. The calm, deep stretching of prenatal yoga opened up my body and strengthened many of the muscles that I intuitively knew I would use in the birth. The yoga was also deeply meditative, so it continued to be the most well-rounded exercise as my pregnancy progressed.

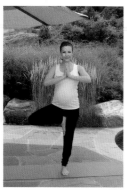
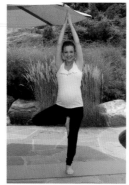
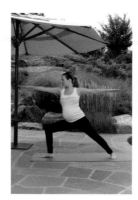
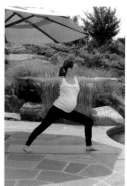

busy body

Not everyone has the luxury of time. Going to a yoga class or to the gym can easily eat up two or more hours of a day, so if that is not feasible for you, find other ways of getting exercise. If you love yoga but don't have the time to go three times a week, commit to going at least once a week, and then make up the other times with quick walks and stretching at home. Ask your yoga teacher which postures are best to do daily, and then try to practice those on your own when you get up or before you go to bed.

If you're a Pilates girl, you can keep up that practice, as there are all kinds of prenatal Pilates courses available. And if you have never done Pilates before, now is a great time to start, since Pilates focuses quite a bit on core strength and works wonders to reshape the body once the baby is born. Sit-ups and crunches are not recommended in the second trimester, because as the uterus grows, its weight can compress blood vessels leading to your heart, and the concern is that this might deprive your developing baby of needed oxygen. Also, lying flat on your back for too long can sometimes lead to lightheadedness, dizziness, nausea and vomiting, as the uterus can also slow blood flow to your brain in this position.

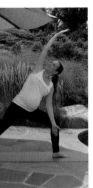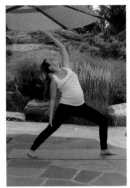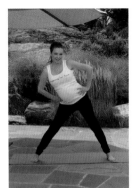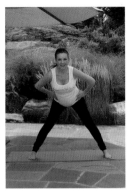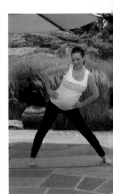

Running and jogging are both perfectly acceptable during this trimester, as long as you do them in moderation. Wear a heart-rate monitor, and try to keep your heart rate under 140 beats per minute, because too rigorous a workout for the rest of the body can divert blood flow to those areas potentially reducing blood flow (or oxygen delivery) to the uterus and your developing baby. Also remember that as your uterus grows, your center of gravity shifts, so balance might start to feel a bit off, which means consider only running or jogging on flat ground. Check in with your doctor about how often it is okay for you to work out.

Finally, remember that as your joints become looser, you are at a greater risk for sprains and strains, so your stretching, warming up, and cooling down will be just as vital as the workout itself. Don't skimp on the details here, as every breath and motion counts.

Remember that exercise during your second trimester not only keeps your metabolism in check but will also help you sleep at night, if insomnia has been an issue. Physical activity in general will only make your pregnancy that much healthier and smoother. Don't be afraid to get creative about how you move—just make sure you do it!

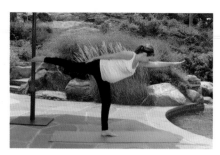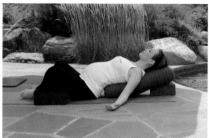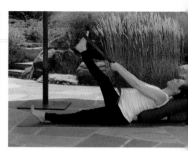

Dancing, for example, is a phenomenal way of getting full-body exercise without having to leave your own home. Fire up the music that gets you moving the most, crank the volume, and let yourself dance. Get your groove on with no holds barred. Throw your arms up in the air and wave them like you just don't care! Dance until you sweat. Babies love dancing in or outside the womb, so you may as well get the party started sooner rather than later.

The absolute best pregnancy exercise is undoubtedly swimming, a low-impact activity that has excellent cardiovascular benefits. There are many reasons why swimming is a favorite for many pregnant women: First of all, you feel lighter in the water, so movement becomes more fluid and less awkward, your joints feel less pressure, your aches are relieved, and your entire body gets a workout. It feels endlessly cleansing, and it's entirely safe.

Most gyms have indoor pools, which are the perfect exercise refuge during the winter; if you are going to swim outdoors, make sure you cover up with sunblock. It's also important to know that the breaststroke is considered the safest for pregnant moms, as it requires little movement of the torso and likewise works both the upper and lower extremities. It also helps to counteract strain in the back due to the weight of pregnancy.

If you want a little more dynamic exercise, however, consider water workouts such as prenatal aqua aerobics or aqua exercise. Aqua aerobics has most of the fat-burning and endurance-building qualities of land-based aerobics without the high-impact pounding

JET-SET MAMA

Think of your second trimester as a perfect opportunity to indulge in some of the little things you are itching to do—like getting away for some good old-fashioned rest and relaxation. Assuming your doctor approves it, this is a great time to plan a romantic getaway and take a serious breather before the frenzy of the third trimester and birth—just as long as you take the necessary precautions and really think your holiday through.

Start by picking a place that makes sense for a pregnancy, a destination that isn't too remote and where there won't be too many diversions and physical exertion—a place where all you have to do is *nothing* ...

Obtain the names of local ob-gyns you can contact should any problem arise, and when you pack, gear up with plenty of prenatal supplements, sunscreen, antibacterial wipes to clean public bathroom seats, any creams or lotions you're using to treat itchiness or prevent stretch marks, and any herbs, teas, pain relievers, and/or medications you're taking for any other ailments, such as gassiness or heartburn.

When booking a flight, make sure the airline knows you're pregnant, and request a seat in the aisle so you can get up easily whenever you need to. Take snacks on the plane with you, since you never know what (or how often) you will be fed while in flight. On the plane and when you arrive, double your intake of fluids, because travel can be very dehydrating.

Have your medical records in your purse at all times, and that includes relevant insurance documents just in case anything happens while you are away. But more than anything, relax and enjoy this stretch of personal time that will feel sacred as things progress toward the birth. Use the time to think deeply about what kind of mother you would like to be.

It is also a good idea when traveling to get up out of your seat (car, train, or plane) and walk around for a few minutes every hour or so. This will help your circulation by pumping the blood out of your legs, preventing a blood clot from developing, and, more importantly, preventing a pulmonary embolus, which is a blood clot that develops in the deep veins of the leg.

that can be injurious while pregnant. If you're self-conscious about being in a bathing suit, try to remember that this is probably the only time in your life when you are *supposed* to look big. Embrace it, and go out and get yourself an adorable maternity suit in a color that makes you happy.

Finally, no schedule is too busy for a few sets of Kegels (see "The Super Vagina," page 50), which can be done anytime, anywhere. Think of your vagina right now as an Olympic athlete in training for the performance of her life. If you do nothing else, do your Kegels!

beauty and the bump

I won't lie: As far as style goes, the fourth month can be dicey. If you're showing already, you've crossed over. You're officially pregnant to the world. Congratulations! But for many of us, at this point in our term, just barely past the first trimester, we look, frankly, fat. Since I did not tell people until well into my fifth month, I was forced to become a costume designer, each outfit an exercise in chic camouflaging. In the end I found many ways to beat the bulge.

bump wrangling

So what if your favorite skinny jeans won't button . . . even if you lie on your bed and squirm around in them. Just let them go for now, hang them up, and make them the motivating force for your diet and exercise regimen postpartum. Know that your buns will one day again grace the perfect seat of those jeans, and when they do, you will again be proud of them. In the interim, there are a million other ways to enhance your beauty.

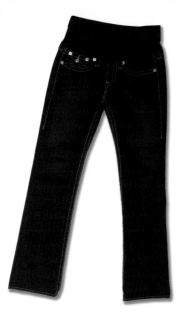

You can continue to look glam and have fun with your style even if there is more of you now than you're used to. Wearing a great-looking pair of jeans with an expandable waist can go a long way toward making women feel stylish again, and with great maternity designs by hip companies like Paige and Habitual, you can continue to rock the jeans look.

Of course, there are other secrets: I found a little miracle in the body-shaping tank on www.yummietummie.com, which holds in your stomach and sides with a microfiber panel in the midsection, perfect to hide those unruly bumps and lumps.

focus on the face

If you want to divert attention away from your midsection, focus on your face. This is a great time to play with styles and techniques you have never tried before. Don't be afraid to tap into your inner diva. Let yourself play. If you've never done the dramatic smoky eye, now is the time. Or get creative with color, and scope out looks that are sexy and smoldering. Get some magazines, tear out looks that appeal to you, and try duplicating them at home. In my first book, *¡Belleza!: Lessons in Lipgloss and Happiness*, I explore all kinds of makeup styles and beauty tips; take a look for yourself, and experiment with new ways of doing your makeup. Or go to a makeup counter and have a makeover. Why not? For the next few months, girlfriend, it's your show. Dare to be a star.

Pampering your skin is another way of keeping the focus on that pretty face, where your natural glow will already be working its magic. If your doctor approves it, try having monthly facials (many spas actually offer prenatal facials, avoiding any glycolics, acids, or peelings); just make sure that all the products used are organic. Go out and buy eye cream. If you are lucky enough to live near the ocean, there is nothing like a daily dip in the sea to make the skin more luminous and clean. Treat your skin like a baby itself; nurture it with all kinds of love.

Use sunscreen every day to avoid patchiness, as the hormonal flux can cause the mela-tonin in the face to group up. Be vigilant about the sunscreen—your skin is scared.

BRINGING SEXY BACK

Another benefit of entering the second trimester is that your libido might kick back into high gear. In my first trimester, with the rampant and recurring pukes, my personal mission was to simply survive every day, and sex was the last thing on my mind. At the same time, strangely, I felt like the sexiest woman on earth. I began to notice that men look at pregnant women like a wolf looking at sheep, which confirms that the glow is not to be underrated. By the fourth month I felt much better, and I moved into my pregnancy with more grace; in that space I found a sexy femininity that lent itself to great fun in the bedroom. I knew that my hormones were still at full throttle, affecting my moods and my body, and I allowed myself to go with the flow of what I was feeling. In this trimester you might start to feel juicier, more alive, even insatiable. Go with those feelings, and see them as a gift.

Though second-trimester sex can be as tender as anything, you will likely have to allay your partner's fears about "the big-headed monster." By that I mean the universal anxiety that most men have of traumatizing the fetus with the presence of their penis. Tell your partner to relax, tell him that your baby wants you to love one another, that it's part of the program. Better yet, use your powers of seduction and show the man how it is done.

Getting your hair styled is another great way to direct attention away from your belly. The truth is, big hair levels out the scope of the belly. And let's face it, when you're properly coiffed, you feel beautiful. There is just something so crisp and polished about a woman with a gorgeously styled head of hair. It's the perfect thing to treat yourself to when you are feeling pudgy rather than pregnant. Get a blowout. Get an up-do. You'll feel terrific and look terrific, too. But be warned: You are going to want to change your hair at the end of the second trimester. You'll be bored, you'll want a change. *Don't do it!* Remember that you are under the influence of your hormones.

bump-wear 201

In the second trimester I lived in long, open, Lycra-cotton dresses with a tank top underneath. It was so freeing, all that fresh air ventilating through the dress at all times. It was heavenly in the face of those insane, hot hormonal flashes.

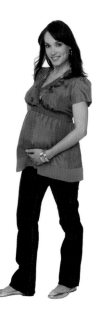

But when it comes to fashion at this point in the game, having lots of interesting tops will really be the key. Think tunics, empire cuts, long T-shirts, men's-style button-downs, cashmere V-necks in every color, sweaters, hoodies, you name it.

Have as many tops as possible, so that you can worry less about the bottom. As you get bigger, you can start to take advantage of some of the slouchier, baggier styles, which are fashionable these days.

Dark colors in long silhouettes are also good choices for obscuring new curves. Long sweaters and vests are versatile and work marvelously over tights, leggings, or skinny jeans (if you can still squeeze yourself into them, God bless you). Cute A-line dresses over tights with boots look fun and feminine and are great in winter, and an oversize cashmere sweater over a pair of leggings is a perfect cozy, sexy look. Here are some chic celeb samples.

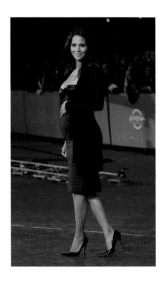
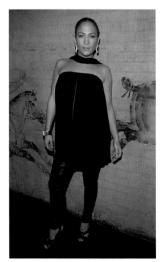
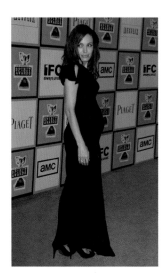

I'm of the school that says that when you are pregnant, you cannot have enough cashmere. Ensconce yourself in as much cashmere as possible—no matter what you're wearing, it always feels good to throw on a soft, luscious shawl. Sweater dresses are also incredibly comfortable and can cover up the bump gracefully while keeping everybody warm 'n' yummy.

Finally, trade in your high-heeled boots for sturdier motorcycle boots, which look great with maternity jeans, casual dresses, and leggings alike. Boots have become the

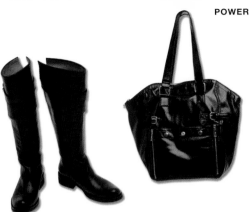

must-have perennial accessory for all women, pregnant or not, and are wearable through spring, summer, and fall. You can get really creative pairing boots with funky tights in bright colors, or hand-knit hosiery, which helps streamline the legs when everything else seems to be growing by the day.

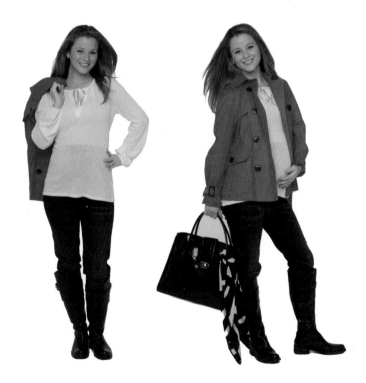

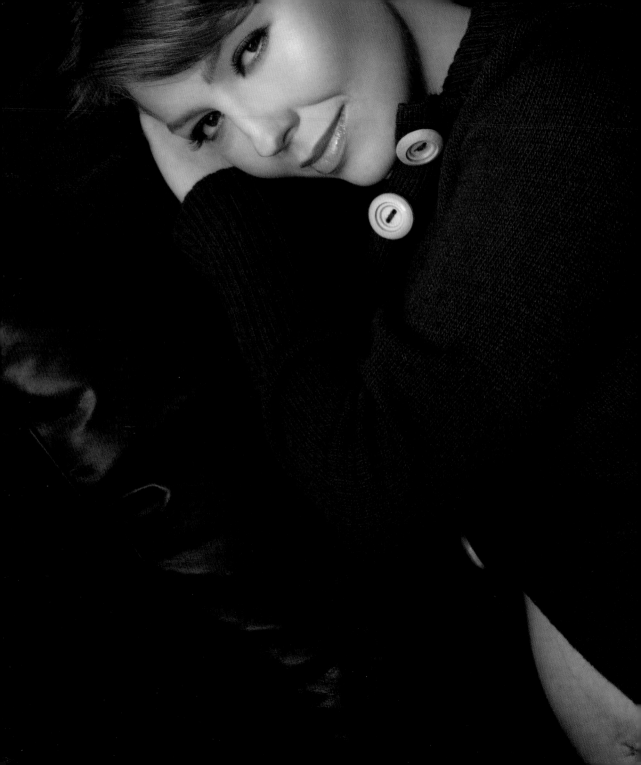

chapter 3: *living large*

THIRD TRIMESTER: WEEKS 28–40/MONTHS 7–9

If you were lucky enough to sail through the second trimester—bump out, energy up, and eyes bright—and you now feel victorious and ready for anything, be grateful. This is exactly the kind of spirit and attitude that you will want and need as things get (literally) heavier entering the seventh month. On the other hand, if you did not feel so hot the last few months, do whatever it takes to toughen up, because the next phase will demand your all in every way.

Even though this trimester continues to be dominated by how much your body is physically changing, and the logistics and administration mobilized for giving birth, this time also provides a profound opportunity for you to connect mentally with the prospect of soon getting to meet the baby you have been devoutly serving and quietly adoring.

I remember one morning, around my thirtieth week, looking down at my belly and bursting into a hysterical and unstoppable fit of laughter, a maniacal cackle replete with tears and heaving. It was a bizarre moment of euphoria and anxiety that tickled me everywhere, making the soon-to-be reality of motherhood seem very tangible. I thought about all the other pregnant women around the world having parallel borderline-hysterical moments, and in that instant it became clear to me that the third trimester would be the final frontier, a raw initiation into the ranks of universal womanhood that I sometimes thought I'd never reach. But there I was, and I was ready.

In this section, as you continue to gather strength to face the rest of the term head-on, we will explore what it means to stay tough, drawing on the powers of looking and feeling great, some basic planning, and an unwavering positive outlook. We'll go over the nuts and bolts of what your body is going through, what it will need, and how your baby is really coming into her own. We'll review checklists, logistics, and planning tips in preparation for the fourth trimester, because while the third trimester is critical mass in *your world*, it is also the time to get set for the fourth trimester, which is when your *baby* will be home. In sum, the third trimester is a juggling act like no other, one that will ask you to be patient, strong, resilient, intentional, and brave. And to that I say, *welcome the challenge* to be this fierce.

dealing with discomforts

Let's be real: By the seventh month and onward, things become more intense. Because you are carrying around a lot more weight, there will be more discomforts. Typically, pregnant women complain of pelvic pressure, inner thigh pain, and sometimes a vaginal shooting pain from "the baby" pressing on nerves. You will become an expert wrangler of simultaneous discomforts and a seasoned master of endurance.

For me, the serious juggling act began with what I like to call "the curse of the dragon"— bouts of acid reflux that would leave me feeling like I'd been spewing flames for hours. I was advised to sleep in a more "sitting up" position, which seemed to help, until I realized that going through the night like that was causing sciatica, a compression of the sciatic nerve that causes pain in the back, legs, and feet. Just to keep things lively, this caused me to have restless leg syndrome, a common symptom of pregnancy in which the legs become tingly and jumpy, often during the night, which of course brought on my good friend insomnia . . . just what I needed.

My point is that sometimes the kinks do not seem to end and instead pile up and frazzle you. In these moments, try to meet the discomfort with your strength, and know deeply that each nuisance and tribulation is one step closer to feeling a healthy, warm newborn asleep in your arms.

Now more than ever you are going to feel like you are carrying a *baby*. You will feel its weight, you will start to understand its humanness more clearly, you might even smirk when you think about what his little personality is like in there. You may also start to feel like you're running out of space inside your womb. You simply have to trust that your body knows what it's doing and have faith that the last few months will allow for the needed expansion. As that growth continues, you will feel the baby moving with greater strength and frequency, which can be a thrilling diversion in a moment of extreme pain or fatigue. See your baby's kicks as his way of telling you that everything is as it should be.

My navel popped out around this time, and I distinctly remember having an itchy sensation in my abdomen. The dark line, called the linea negra, from my belly button to my pubic bone also became more pronounced, and by the time I got to the eighth month, I started to feel Braxton Hicks contractions, which help get the uterus in practice for its future work during labor. I also had to urinate more often, a result of my baby "dropping," adding more pressure on my bladder.

Many of the symptoms you feel now may be amplified versions of sensations you've been feeling since the first trimester, or some entirely new things might crop up. Because every woman's chemistry is unique, the way we present symptoms (or not) will vary. Following is a list of symptoms that you will likely encounter if you have not already. Even though you may find yourself nodding yes to each ailment in this long list, take comfort in the fact that this means you are having a *totally normal* pregnancy, and none of these items (despite their discomfort) are necessarily cause for alarm. (See pages 24 and 84 for tips to treat many of these ailments.)

❋ Appetite changes

❋ Bleeding gums

❋ Clumsiness

❋ Heartburn, flatulence, bloating

❋ Hemorrhoids

❋ Increased fatigue

❋ Increased vaginal discharge

❋ Insomnia

❋ Leaky nipples

❋ Digestive issues

❋ Headaches, dizziness

❋ Leg cramps or pain

❋ Overheating

❋ Pelvic pressure or pain

❋ Rib pain

❋ Stronger fetal activity

❋ Swollen feet and ankles (edema)

Bring up any serious or chronic issues with your healthcare provider, and certainly mention things that seem out of the ordinary or that seem to really restrict you. Since you will likely be seeing more of your doctor in the final months of your pregnancy, use these golden opportunities to put on the table whatever you'd like to address.

final screening and testing

By week 28, you should have a glucose screen for gestational diabetes (see "Other Second-Trimester Tests," page 89). If you fail your glucose screen don't panic. Remember that this is only a screening test and most women who fail this test do not necessarily have gestational diabetes. You will, however, have to take a more detailed second test, which you will most likely pass. If you fail the second test, it means you are having trouble metabolizing sugar during your pregnancy and will have to go on a special diet and check your blood sugars during the pregnancy.

At weeks 35–37, you may be offered a Group B strep infection screening, which looks for a bacterium in the vagina that, though not necessarily harmful to you, can be serious if passed to your baby during the birth.

Any time after twenty-eight weeks, you may have an external nonstress test to monitor the fetal heart rate and heart rate patterns. Some mothers feel that fetal heart monitoring is not necessary and interferes with the natural birthing process, while other women see the test as ultimately reassuring. Before you decide, it's important to know what your options are. Electronic heart monitoring can be done during pregnancy, labor, and delivery. There are two types:

External monitoring is used to listen to your baby's heartbeat as well as to monitor the frequency of your contractions. Your baby's heartbeat can be heard with a special stethoscope, but more commonly it is monitored by using a flat sensor held in place by an elastic belt placed around your belly. This sensor uses reflected sound waves (ultrasound) to keep track of your baby's heart rate. Another sensor also placed on your belly is used to measure the frequency and duration of your contractions.

Internal monitoring is reserved for labor and delivery; it can be done only after your cervix has dilated and your amniotic sac has ruptured. When internal fetal heart rate monitoring is performed, a thin wire (electrode) is inserted through your vagina and cervix into your uterus. The electrode is then attached to your baby's scalp. If internal contraction monitoring is performed, a small tube that measures the strength of uterine contractions will be inserted through the vagina and cervix into the uterus next to your baby. Your baby's heartbeat may be heard as a beeping sound or printed out on a chart.

Internal monitoring is said to be more accurate than external monitoring for keeping track of both fetal heart rate and contractions.

At around week 28, you may be given a shot to prevent what is known as "Rh sensitization." Each of us has a blood type that is either Rh positive or Rh negative, meaning that our blood cells either have the Rh antigen on their surface (Rh positive) or do not (Rh negative). If the fetus has the Rh antigens on its blood cell surface but the mother does not, her immune system, recognizing the fetal blood as a substance not her own, might read the fetus as a foreign invader and attempt to fight it. Even worse, it could jeopardize future pregnancies. For these reasons this shot, known as RhoGAM, is given as a preventative measure. The first dose is administered at twenty-eight weeks, and a second is given within a day or two after the baby's birth.

By now your baby is gaining up to half a pound a week, and the temporary protective hair called lanugo is starting to fall off. Tiny fingernails and toenails are now present, and some babies also start to grow their real hair around this time. Though the lungs and brain are still immature at the beginning of the trimester, by the ninth month, radical growth and development will have occurred.

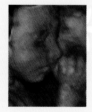

By the eighth month (28 weeks), your baby is 18–19 inches long and weighs 4–5 pounds.

p is for prioritize

The last three months of your term are your chance to lock in some of the basics for your quickly approaching delivery. Remember that typically the birth can occur two weeks before or after the due date. If you're at seven months, you will notice that all of a sudden the prospect of giving birth in two months and two weeks starts to feel very real. On the flip side, the weeks may also start to seem interminable now, as you struggle to lug your heavy, sweaty, uncomfortable self around town, huffing and puffing, waiting and wondering. But trust me, time will start to fly, and you'll want to have all your ducks lined up when things start to really get cooking.

the place

If you have not yet decided on a birthing center, now is the time to get serious about the research. The sooner you have a hospital or birthing center in place or secured arrangements to deliver in your own home, the better (see also "Location, Location, Location," page 21, for a refresher about your options). Many hospitals offer preregistration, which speeds up the check-in process—and I can guarantee that if you're in active labor, the last thing you will have the head for is paperwork.

the plan

Think of your birthing plan as your wish list for what you envision your delivery to be. My own consisted of some very specific items (barring any complications), including getting to look at a mirror at the peak of the birth itself—when the baby's head comes out—and the chance for my husband to cut my cord. The only time this cannot occur is if the cord is wrapped tightly around the neck when the baby's head is delivered. Then, as a matter of safety, the obstetrician should do it.

I also asked that my baby be given to me at the moment of her birth so that we could experience instantaneous skin-to-skin contact. I wanted her to feel me before she felt anything else, and I wanted her to know that I was still right here. I see it as the mother of all meetings. It was also my hope to be able to deliver the baby vaginally, and I was even up for going without an epidural (until the twenty-eighth hour of my labor, when I came to my senses and begged for the drugs, then kissed the hands of the man who administered them to me). I didn't want to have a C-section if I could avoid it. I wanted to connect with the natural process of giving birth. I kept thinking of a C-section as cheating, even though I would have had one in a heartbeat if it were necessary.

The point is that you should think about all of the variables that are being thrown at you and try to make decisions *starting now* about what you envision for yourself. Be your own advocate. Don't assume that you are just another woman on deck for a birth, to be told what to do, how to do it, and when to do it. Start thinking about how you would like your birthing experience to be. If you're not sure about what belongs in a birthing plan, here are some considerations:

✳ Being able to walk around while in labor

✳ Circumcision, if it's a boy

✳ Eating or drinking during labor

✳ Filming or taking photographs of the birth

✳ Having an episiotomy or not

✳ Having music, lighting, or other atmospheric elements in place

✳ Holding and/or breast-feeding your baby right away

✳ The presence of your partner and other relatives or friends

✳ The use of a mirror, so you can see the birth

✳ The use of synthetic hormones to induce contractions

✳ What position you want to be in when you deliver

✳ Which visitors are permitted and when

✳ Who cuts the cord, and when (some women want to meet their baby first)

the practice

Today, being informed about birthing is widely accessible not only through literature but also through birthing classes. Each type of class espouses its own attitude and approach to birth and birthing, and you will inevitably learn something about how to prepare for, endure, and make the most of your experience at whichever class you choose to attend. At the very least, you will learn about the process and get a sense of what your labor and delivery options may be.

You might enroll in a course that teaches Lamaze, a birthing style that involves intentional breathing and concentration. Another birthing technique is the Bradley Method, a natural approach that emphasizes the powerful and supportive role that a partner can play in the childbirth—so that the mother will not require drugs or surgery. In fact, there are many different natural birthing styles that espouse medication-free birth and teach visualizations, hypnosis, and pain-management exercises as coping mechanisms to get through the experience. The sooner you begin this preparatory work, the better armed you will be when push comes to shove (literally!).

If you are considering breastfeeding, you might want to enroll in a breastfeeding class or meet with a lactation specialist (see also "Engorgement," page 172, for more about breastfeeding) who can guide you and help you prepare yourself (and your breasts) for that process. See these last three months as your chance to soak up as much information as possible, because once the baby is born, you will not want to be bothered.

the people

If you have chosen to work with a doula, now is the time to make that selection, too, not only because the good ones book up fast but because you will want your doula's insights and advice about preparation early on, not to mention the chance to really forge a connection with her before the moment of truth comes. (See "I ❤ My Doula," on the facing page, about my own personal doula experience.) For more advice on selecting a labor coach— be it a midwife, your partner, or your mom, see "Build Your Dream Team," page 17.

If you fear you might not have adequate help from family, friends, or your partner, you might consider a baby nurse (see "Keep Building Your Dream Team," page 82). The point is, if you anticipate needing any extra help whatsoever, keep the hiring process moving along. Trust me: You will not want to be worrying about this after you've given birth.

Finally, when you are thinking about the people on your team, include the obstetrics nurses in the hospital (if applicable) who will attend to you, and consider bringing them each a small gift, such as a box of chocolates, as a gesture of goodwill, knowing that you will be dealing with them intimately while you are in the hospital. Nothing wrong with starting out on everyone's good side.

the postpartum

After the beautiful storm that is labor and delivery, there will be a calm. You will find yourself in a hospital room—or in your own bedroom for home births—totally exhausted, and you will want what you want. That may mean fudge popsicles for one person, the Beatles' *White Album* for another, or cashmere blankets for someone else. We all know what our favorite comforts are, be they music, chocolate, a certain scent, a special pillow, whatever—only you know what yours is. A good friend of mine brought me pink sheets, a robe, towels, and roses; she personalized that sterile room for me, and it made all the difference. Think about the comforts you might want after you've given birth (excluding things like cigarettes and martinis), and make even these details part of the cultivation of your own unique, personal experience. Add your comfort items to the overnight bag you're taking to the hospital or birthing center (see "It's in the Bag," page 141), and have the bag at the ready in case you go into labor early.

the pediatrician

As you get closer to delivery, you should select your *baby's* doctor, since you will want a pediatrician to check the baby as soon as possible. Research your choices. Referrals are always the best way to go, so begin by talking to your own doctor, friends, and family members. You can also visit the Web site of the American Academy of Pediatrics at www.aap.org/referral. As with selecting your own doctor, you'll want to keep your healthcare insurance at the forefront of your consideration (see "The Insurance Issue," page 19).

the partner

The third trimester is also a good time to begin deciding what the role of your partner will be in the birth. You may have already discussed this and have a clear sense of it, or you may be clueless. In my case, we decided that the role of my partner (besides adoring, supporting, and pampering me with every cell in his body) would be to film the birth, not only so that we could archive the moment but so that he would have something tangible to focus on, which I knew I would need (wink) to keep the calm in the room (see "Partner's Part," page 20).

I ❤ MY DOULA

From the moment I came across the word "doula," I just adored it. I quickly learned that women all over the world give birth with the help of a doula, or someone who steps into the role of birth-coach/birth-partner with infinitely more calm and savvy than say . . . um . . . an overly nervous spouse or an annoyingly protective grandma-to-be. The doula takes charge as your advocate for a totally harmonious experience as you prepare for birthing, through the delivery itself, and even postpartum. My husband being squeamish, and my mother the kind of woman who gets panicky when direct sunlight hits my face, I knew I needed a second-in-command to step in with certitude when things got going.

I asked my ob-gyn for a recommendation, knowing that the doula ultimately cannot be in the way of the doctor; I needed to make sure that everyone would get along. By inquiring with my doctor, I knew I would get a referral for someone that he felt good about, which would help keep the energy in the birthing room positive. I learned that my doula had helped in more than two hundred births; she clearly knew what she was doing, and that alone gave me tremendous comfort.

Each woman will have her own ideas about what she'd like the birthing experience to be, and so your doula should share and support your vision. You might want to work with someone who is high energy, who will actively motivate you to rise above the pain into the joy of motherhood, or you might need the silent touch of a doula to center your awareness and help you quiet your mind. I interviewed five doulas and settled on someone with a fairly neutral energy, a woman who would support me when I was at the peak of my contractions, who would remind me to drink a lot of water, who would massage my hips in the right way.

During labor, when I got to the point that I could not deal with the pain, she calmly took my hand and suggested a short walk, knowing that exactly in that moment walking would alleviate me. She knew that I wanted to experience as much of the labor as possible at home and not be rushed to a hospital, and having her at my side on those very last days gave me the confidence to undergo much of the labor in the comfort and quiet of my own home. The day I went to the hospital she drew a bath for me with lavender, lit the candles, and got the music going. I stepped in, and we just talked. I managed to stay in my house relaxing for two more hours before rushing to the hospital. Those two hours were sacred to me, and just for that my doula was everything.

heads up: the signs

As you move into the later phases of your term, there are some key moments, also known as pre-labor, that signal the birth's closeness. Though the early labor signs may not be too pretty, embrace them as tangible evidence that everything is moving in the right direction—and use them to plan and mobilize accordingly.

About two to four weeks before the birth, your baby will "drop" into your pelvis, getting into position for its grand exit. This is also known as "lightening" or "engagement." You might notice this change visibly, because your belly feels lower, or because you are urinating a whole lot more due to the new pressure on your bladder.

A less-than-lovely phenomenon that you might notice several weeks before the delivery is the mucus plug, a thick, gooey material that keeps your cervix sealed during the pregnancy and starts to thin out as the cervix begins the initial phases of dilation. Some women pass it, some women don't, and either way, it is not necessarily an indicator that the birth is happening on that day. If you do see it, just know that it's a sign that everything is as it should be. The same is true for bloody discharge (also referred to as "bloody show"), which is also just the cervix doing its thing in preparation and transition for the birth. If your discharge appears as very bright red, to play it safe, contact your doctor, as this can sometimes indicate complications with the placenta.

Contractions are the events we're all taught to look out for. The Braxton Hicks contractions that may have started in spurts during the second trimester will likely increase in intensity, and once the actual contractions start happening regularly, you will know you are beginning your labor. These may feel like intense menstrual cramps or a really upset stomach.

Your water (or amniotic sac) breaking is another signpost that the delivery is near. Don't panic; just get in touch with your doctor or midwife (and doula, if you have one). Calmly follow their instructions, and, in the meantime, keep the vagina as clean as possible to prevent infection.

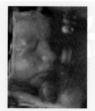

By the ninth month (33 weeks), your baby is 19–21 inches long and weighs 6–9 pounds.

Even as you navigate all of the physical details of the birthing process, try to also see these last three months as your own inner prep time to herald in a whole new era of your life. As you continue to juggle the emotional and physical world of pregnancy while it kicks into high gear, keep this notion in the back of your mind.

lead with your heart

With so much happening physically during this trimester, the mental stuff can easily get swept aside. But now more than ever is the time to work out the mind kinks, those subtle but pesky negativities that creep up and try to sabotage our peace of mind. The last trimester of your pregnancy is nothing short of holy: It is your time to redefine your standards of wellness—physically *and* mentally—so that your baby can come into this world totally suffused in positivity and health. Your mental state will impact the rest of your body, and a negative outlook will definitely add unneeded stress and tension to what will already be a very challenging couple of months. I found that verbalizing every little thing that was bothering me was the most therapeutic way to go; somehow, by acknowledging all of my angst with words, it would be released from me and could not brew further or remain stuck inside.

With everything going on, it may seem impossible to maintain the razor-sharp focus you need to stay cool. You may be feeling a world of emotions, ranging from excitement and curiosity to being ready for the whole mess to be over. Your dream life may be taking on some *Rosemary's Baby*–like proportions, freaking you out well into the morning. You may start to feel like some kind of alien, impatiently waddling around, exasperated and ragged. You may feel all these things at once or none of them at all. But quite naturally, for many women, some anxiety will start to build, and inevitably the questions will begin their circular parade through the mind: *How painful is that first contraction going to be? How will I know when to go to the hospital? What will the first night be like? How will I know how to understand what my baby wants? Will I be able to breastfeed? How will I know how to bathe her? Who will tell me if I am doing it right? How will I clean her tiny eyes, and how will I calm her cries, and more important, how will I know which are cries of hunger and which are shrieks of exhaustion?*

I remember also starting to get a sense of claustrophobia during this time, imagining my little girl, like a little tamale, all stuffed together and wrapped up tightly in her little sac. And then I would immediately think to myself, if she can sense what I am feeling, she very well might start to feel claustrophobic herself. That final thought would cause me to shake off the feelings and relax. Prenatal claustrophobia is a common sensation that many pregnant women experience—if you suffer from this ailment as well, try to accept it as one more layer to the brilliant but complex process of birthing.

Just as in the first two trimesters, I diligently continued my visualization exercises, doing them at the same time every day to help me stay on track. They were my salvation on some of the days when I felt the worst. The intention of connecting with my baby daily proved stronger than any pain or discomfort. Making the most out of one's pregnancy through deep awareness of the mind-body connection is an idea that became like an anchor for me during the most challenging moments.

If you are not the kind of person who can meditate or even relax, here's another suggestion: Distract yourself. Online shopping, for example, became a fantastic in-bed diversion for me when I wasn't feeling tip-top. From my house in New York, I would phone a long-distance friend, then we'd both open up our laptops and scour the Internet together for adorable little outfits, comparing, giggling, anticipating, and imagining. You will begin to see all of those sweet little shoes and blankets and toys, and they'll remind you of the interminable world of cuteness that is about to come, which is all you may need to pull you through your funk. Start shopping for the nursery, or begin a baby shower registry (see "Baby Showers," page 143, for a list of common registry items).

Another way to productively distract yourself is to think about naming the baby. One consideration is the *meaning* of names. For example, in Spanish there are names that have blatantly positive meanings, like Luz (light) or Sol (sun). But there are also some overly dramatic names, such as Soledad (solitude). You might also consider nicknames and languages: In our case we wanted a name that would sound right in English and Spanish, so both of our families could easily pronounce it.

I had always wanted a daughter named Sabrina, though I never knew its meaning. But with a little research, I discovered that Sabrina means "princess." Later I came across the name Sakaë, which means "prosperity" in Japanese, and the two names—Sabrina Sakaë—rang in my ears. My husband and I loved the two names together, as they made her independent from us, her very own person.

table for two: what to eat in the third trimester

As you edge toward delivery, nutrition remains as crucial to the baby as it has been since the beginning, and perhaps even more so. Research and studies have shown that protein intake during the third trimester actually helps to promote optimal fetal brain development, so if you haven't been taking in the requisite three servings daily, now is the time to start getting serious about it (see "Protein," page 96).

If time or lack of energy is an issue (and both commonly are at this point in the pregnancy), consider making foods and meal selections that freeze well, so you (or your partner) can make a week's worth on a Sunday night and nibble all week. Think stews, soups, casseroles, and even things like macaroni and cheese, which, by the way, tastes just as good with whole wheat noodles and low-fat cheese (see the recipe, "The Smart Mac," page 130). You can also make large batches of things like brown rice, which Eastern medicine calls the most perfectly balanced food, or quinoa, which is a great source of protein—both of which can last for several days in your fridge. By the way, this freezing business will come in handy during the postpartum period, when cooking will be the last thing on your mind.

Something else that is likely to start happening in this trimester is what I like to call "sloppy permissiveness," also known as "I'm-gonna-eat-that-hot-fudge-sundae-cause-why-the-hell-not?" It's that liberty that very pregnant women decide to give themselves, thinking that those calories will hide somewhere in that big belly. This is a mistake, as it will only delay getting your figure back after the birth. So go easy . . .

THE SMART MAC

Here's another one of Esther Blum's recipes that you can tweak to make less fattening and more nutritious. Just make a big ol' batch and freeze the rest!

2 tablespoons olive oil, plus more for greasing

2 tablespoons all-purpose flour (or whole wheat flour)

1½ cups nonfat milk, hot but not boiling

1½ cups freshly grated Parmesan cheese (look for a low-fat variety)

Salt

Freshly ground black pepper

¾ pound macaroni noodles (or whole wheat macaroni)

¼ cup grated sharp Cheddar cheese (look for a low-fat variety)

¼ cup bread crumbs (or whole wheat bread crumbs)

Preheat the oven to 375°F and lightly brush a 2-quart casserole dish with olive oil. Bring a large pot of water to boil. In a 2-quart saucepan, whisk the olive oil and flour together over medium heat and cook for about 2 minutes. Slowly whisk in the hot milk and simmer, stirring occasionally, for 5 minutes. Stir in the Parmesan cheese and season to taste with salt and pepper, and set aside. Add the macaroni to the boiling water and cook until the pasta is al dente, or according to the box's cooking instructions. Drain the pasta. Pour the macaroni into the prepared casserole dish, immediately pour the mixture over it, and stir to combine. Sprinkle the grated cheese over the top, then sprinkle the bread crumbs over the cheese. Bake, uncovered, for about 30 minutes, or until the edges are bubbling and the top is golden brown. Remove from the oven and let stand for 10 minutes before serving.

WHITE BEAN, KALE, AND ROASTED VEGETABLE SOUP

Here's a recipe from Bon Appétit *magazine that is healthy, hearty, packed with protein and calcium, and perfect to make in large batches and freeze. This soup screams cozy winter goodness!*

Nonstick vegetable oil spray

3 medium carrots, peeled and quartered lengthwise

2 large tomatoes, quartered

1 large onion, cut into 8 wedges

½ small butternut squash, peeled, seeded, and cut lengthwise into ½-inch-thick wedges

6 garlic cloves, unpeeled

1 tablespoon olive oil

Salt and pepper

6 cups (or more) canned vegetable broth

4 cups finely chopped kale

3 large, fresh thyme sprigs

1 bay leaf

One 15-ounce can Great Northern beans, drained

Preheat the oven to 400°F. Spray a rimmed baking sheet with oil spray and arrange all the vegetables (minus the kale) on the sheet. Drizzle with olive oil and sprinkle with salt and pepper. Toss and coat. Bake, stirring occasionally, until the vegetables are brown and tender, about 45 minutes. Transfer the carrots and squash to a work surface and cut into ½-inch pieces; set aside. Peel the garlic cloves; place in a processor. Add tomatoes and onion and puree until almost smooth. Pour ½ cup of broth onto the baking sheet and scrape up any browned bits. Transfer broth and vegetable puree to a large pot. Add 5½ cups of broth, plus kale, thyme, and bay leaf, to the pot; bring to a boil. Reduce heat and simmer uncovered until the kale is tender, about 30 minutes. Add the beans and reserved carrots and squash to the soup. Simmer 8 minutes to blend flavors, adding more broth to soup if necessary. Season with salt and pepper to taste and discard the bay leaf and thyme sprigs. Cover and chill, then simply bring to a simmer before serving.

TOO TIRED TO COOK?

Trust me, I understand that the larger you get, the less inclined you will be to spend time on your feet in the kitchen, but there are little things you can do to keep the right kinds of nutrients coursing through your body. If you feel overwhelmed by exhaustion, as I did, don't overthink your meals. Keep it simple with power-punching breakfasts of instant oatmeal and fresh fruit, and keep your protein kicking with easy snacks like soymilk fruit smoothies and mixed nuts. Make practical choices, such as picking up a fresh rotis- serie chicken, which you can eat for at least two or three days, or commit to making a quick stop for a freshly squeezed veggie juice between errands at least three times a week. You don't even have to think about it, and it takes less than a minute for you to drink up those amazing nutrients.

power on . . . and the art of moving when you feel like a walrus

Some women work out until the very last minute, their massive bellies on their tight little frames looking more like an accessory than a load. If you have the stamina for it, fan- tastic; however, you must consult your doctor and with exercise professionals who are well informed about the pregnant body and relevant fitness risks. The fact is, by the ninth month you should start taking it easy. The amount of weight that you lift and the quantity of the reps need to be modified, so do not take it upon yourself to decide what those numbers should be. If you are working out to the end of your term, remember to stretch

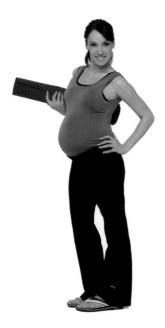

before and after all of your workouts, be more vigilant about keeping your eyes on the clock (and your heart rate) to avoid overexercising, and always cool down after your workout.

By the time I got to the end of my seventh month, exercise was no longer an option for me. All I wanted to be was horizontal. As limber and energized as I felt during my second trimester, my third was like the first one, only I was more tired, fatter, crankier, and less inclined to do anything other than take it easy. But I knew that it was important to keep my body moving, even minimally, to keep up my circulation and avoid swelling in my feet. I also knew that any hard work I put in now would pay off months later, when I would be trying to squirm back into my skinny jeans.

I decided that I would, at the very least, attempt a regimen of easy-to-do, drama-free exercises, the ones you don't even have to leave your bed to do. Leg lifts are one such exercise: Lie on your side, keep your legs straight, and slowly lift and lower the top leg in sets of ten to twenty repetitions. You can also keep a set of 3-pound dumbbells on your bedside table for a few quick sets of bicep and tricep curls, right from bed. Trust me, when you are lugging around a baby in one arm and a stroller and three shopping bags in the other, you'll be glad you worked those guns.

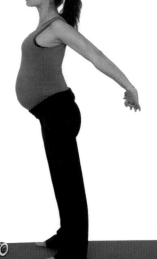

Water aerobics is a great way to lessen the pressure on the joints while at the same time work your muscles. Check both outdoor and indoor pool facilities for classes. Be sure that the person instructing you is trained in what moves and postures are safe during pregnancy and which ones should be avoided.

There are plenty of stretches you can do that don't require tons of physical exertion and will surely keep your joints and muscles nice and flexible. Try to hold these stretches for fifteen to thirty seconds, and remember to take long, slow, deep breaths as you do them.

✳ **Back stretching:** On a soft surface, start on your hands and knees, with knees directly below your hips, hands directly beneath your shoulders, and spine and neck in a relaxed, neutral position. Take a deep inhale and tuck your chin into your chest, drawing your lower abdomen in toward the spine as you round your back like an angry cat. Do at least five sets, and try to hold the pose for at least five to ten seconds.

✳ **Neck stretching:** Sit cross-legged on a soft surface, with your torso upright, shoulders relaxed, and spine straight. With your left hand, gently hold the right side of your head while you reach the opposite hand behind your back. Tilt your head toward your left shoulder until you feel a gentle stretch in the neck, and take deep breaths in that position. Do the same with the right side.

✳ **Full-body stretching:** Begin on your hands and knees, again keeping hands directly beneath shoulders and knees under hips. Slowly straighten your knees, lifting your hips upward, and lower your heels to the ground. Inhale and exhale deeply as you lengthen through the spine. If you can, try to lengthen through your arms, and lower your chest, shifting your weight toward your heels. Try at least five sets, and hold the pose for at least five to ten seconds.

SIMPLY STRETCHING

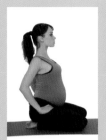

Quad stretch: Start on all fours with a straight back. Slowly lift your torso and come to a sitting position, slowly sitting your buttocks onto your heels until you feel a stretch on the tops of your thighs. Take a deep breath, keeping the spine straight, but relaxed. Hold for about five seconds and release, and do four sets. This is a great precursor for the upcoming hip openers.

Hip opener: Start by sitting upright on the floor with your right leg bent at the knee in front of you, and the left knee bent behind you, holding yourself upright with your straight arms and spine. Take a deep breath and very slowly lean forward, feeling the stretch in the right hip. Hold for about five seconds and do about four sets, on each side. This works well to open the hips and thighs.

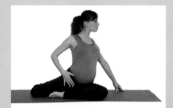

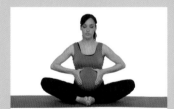

Tailor exercise: Sit on the floor with your knees bent and soles of your feet together, as close to you as possible. Place your hands under your knees and press down with your knees while resisting the pressure with your hands. Count slowly to three, then relax. Place your hands on your belly between sets, and gradually increase the number of reps, with a goal of doing ten per day. The objective is to have the knees go as far to the ground as possible, without bouncing, but trying to push your knees towards the floor. This simple stretch helps strengthen the pelvic, hip, and thigh muscles and also helps relieve lower back pain.

beauty and the bump

I am eternally grateful that the crazy hormone cocktail that swished and swirled in my body, especially during the last three months, didn't make me so loopy that I abandoned my sense of style. I took my commitment to chic to the end of term, knowing that looking my best would help me assert my pride in womanhood, even in the toughest of times. That doesn't mean I was a fully decked-out glamazon at eight months. Quite the contrary: I actually felt more inclined to go with natural looks toward the end of my pregnancy, caring less about hiding it or distracting from it. I was more comfortable and confident with the massive truth that slung right under my very voluptuous breasts. As

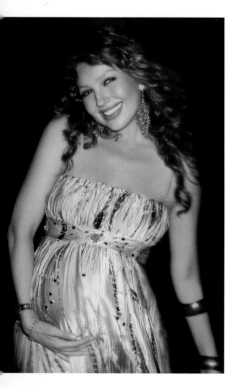

big as I was (and I was really big by the end), I kept feeling beautiful, and I built my style around that aura of confidence. Though I didn't perform a complete makeup job every morning, I tried to at least cover the basics—mascara, blush, and lip gloss—and found that just that touch helped me feel pretty and strong.

The aesthetics of each bump will vary, as each woman carries differently. By this stage, your belly will start to have its own particular shape, depending on the position of your baby, your diet and exercise, and how much weight you've put on.

Because a weighted beach ball has taken over the rest of your body, and pretty much become the first thing people see, now is the time to surrender to it. Fully glorify your pregnancy by wearing that superbump with nothing but pride. Instead of hiding under loose-fitting shirts and baggy pants, wear body-hugging shapes like leggings or tights and clingy tops that happily reveal your ever-curvy shape. I was not afraid to wear a halter top, knowing that a sexy, bare back would be a nice thing to feature, in contrast to the big old belly up in the front.

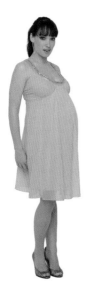 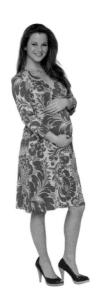 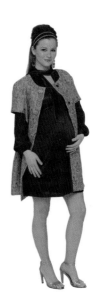

The math may not seem to add up, but it is true: The bigger you are, the prouder you can be of your silhouette. When you are this large, you will be forgiven many things. You will, if only for a moment, be exempt from the perpetual mission to be a rock-hard size 2; you can play with your own comfortable edge of fashion, through color and texture, without feeling the pressures of the magazines or runways. You can truly let go and, in that space of freedom, find ways to rock out and look your best.

Some key changes in your closet can help you through the final stretch. Footwear, for example, becomes essential now. With all the extra weight you are carrying, you may want to consider getting a few pairs of sneakers or other comfortable shoes in a half size larger to accommodate swollen feet and ankles. Say good-bye to your friends Manolo and Jimmy, sniff sniff. Your bra size may have also gone up, for which you may need some new styles and sizes. No big whoop. Just go with the flow, and don't pass judgment on yourself if the changes seem to be coming on too much and a bit too fast. It's all part of the process, and all of us are different.

Some women, for example, develop heavier upper arms as they get bigger, a not-so-fun variable to consider when choosing which top to wear, say, on a hot summer morning. If you feel fleshy in the arm, get yourself an arsenal of tops that cover those parts, like cuts with slenderizing quarter-length sleeves, or a men's-style button-down with sleeves you can casually roll up.

As far as skin care goes, if you haven't already started, it's a good time to start using anti–stretch mark lotions, of which there are tons. In fact, right when you start seeing the first signs of stretch marks or other blemishes, you should start diligently applying the lotions daily. My personal favorites are La Roche-Posay Active C and Mustela, both of which made my skin feel refreshed and supple, and which I continued to use months after my baby was born.

nesting, best thing

You always hear about the whole "nesting" thing, that urge that women (and men, too, in my husband's case) start feeling around this stage to purge and cleanse. I definitely felt it. I wanted to throw out everything in my closets and drawers and refill them with

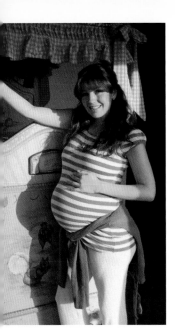

newness and perfection. I felt the impulse to turn my entire world of belongings inside out and start fresh. I understood that it was simply my psyche making room for the next chapter, and I welcomed this impulse to maximize my productivity during this tiring and busy time.

I used this nesting mojo to make shopping lists for fundamental gear, like diapers, car seats, and receiving blankets. (Read on for a complete list of baby basics.) I started to think about the crib and the changing station. I began to browse baby stores, buying clothes I loved. Some of my favorite shopping Web sites are www.giggle.com, www.poshtots. com, and www.petitetresor.com.

I quickly learned to wash the baby clothes with a hypoallergenic soap; I only used green, eco-friendly products for everything from laundry detergent to the cleanser for the breast pump gear. I kept the momentum up as I continued to carve out a space for the baby in our home, physically and mentally.

baby basics

Ready or not, the moment has finally come for you to consider your first round of baby gear, the arsenal of stuff you'll need to have in place before the baby is born. At first the onslaught of warm and fuzzy objects seems totally daunting; I felt like my mind had been invaded by the sounds of squeeze toys and electronic lullabies, their sugary-sweet melodies all starting to sound exactly the same. The list of things to account for seemed so long and annoyingly detailed. I had no idea where to start, or what was crucial. But after some deep breathing, surveying my books, consulting with my sisters and close girlfriends, cross-referencing and consolidating what everyone had to say, I realized that the checklist of the absolute musts is not that daunting at all.

The idea is to not make yourself crazy. A good place to start is thinking about the kind of nursery you want to create for your baby, considering color, mood, and overall aesthetic. The large pieces will be the crib and changing station. My challenge was that I had to decorate three different nurseries for our three homes—one in New York, one in Colorado, and one in Florida—and believe you me, after getting through with the trio, I became a veritable expert.

There are plenty of online resources across the financial spectrum for nursery furniture and accessories. (See "Resources," page 195). At PoshTots, I found an adorable motif of bunnies in its Carrot collection, and the Safari bedding collection from Wendy Bellissimo (www.wendybellissimo.com) is also divine. But you don't have to spend a fortune—basic resources, like www.babiesrus.com and www.buybuybaby.com, will have every single thing you need and more.

Once you have the baby's room theme, or even just a color scheme, making a shopping list for other fundamental things like strollers, car seats, and linens will fall into place easily. The following is a list of the essentials. If you can, have these ready before the baby comes, because once she's here, trust me, you won't have the energy to go shopping. Better yet, register for the items as gift ideas for a baby shower (see "Baby Shower," page 142). For starters, here are some great gift suggestions to think about:

❋ Bedding and towels	❋ Activity gym	❋ Baby books
❋ Bath set	❋ Baby carrier/sling	❋ Picture frames
❋ Bounce seat	❋ Baby monitor	❋ Toys

IT'S IN THE BAG

When the contractions are five minutes apart, you'll be grateful that you—or your partner—don't have to worry about the details. In that typically hectic flurry of excitement and emotion, you will want to know that you have every little thing that you may need. Packing a bag for the hospital absolves you of having to stress about it on the way out the door. Here's a list of things you should pack, though some may be provided by your hospital or birthing center:

* Birth plan
* Breast pads*
* Camera and film or memory card, plus extra battery or charger
* Comfortable labor clothes
* Comfortable robe that you don't mind getting stained
* Favorite snacks and drinks
* Fresh, lemony cologne, something that smells clean and crisp
* Hospital underwear (disposable are best)
* Insurance papers
* iPod loaded with music you like
* Medicated soothing wipes*
* Motrin
* Nursing bra, or other comfy bra

* Personal toiletries
* Sanitary napkins
* Slippers
* Something to read
* Special blanket or pillow
* Special photographs you may want nearby, or images of your spiritual leaders
* Squirt bottle*
* Stool softeners*

FOR BABY:

* Blankets
* Booties or little socks
* Comfy clothing that won't irritate the belly button
* Hat

* See "Dealing with Discomforts . . . and the many untold truths within the secret society," page 164, for the uses of these items.

BABY SHOWER

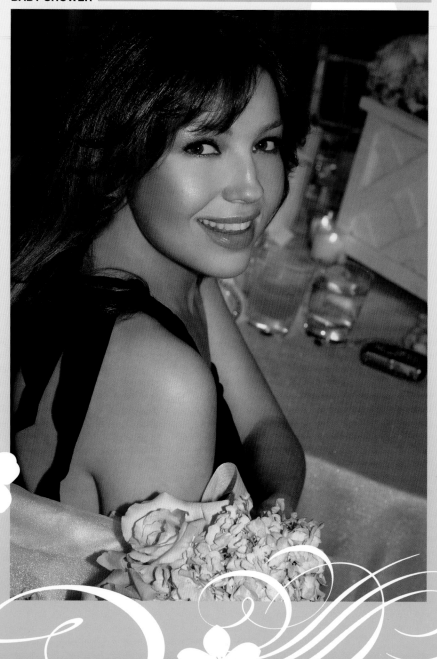

Baby showers—aptly named since they are a time for showering your baby and yourself with love—are typically organized towards the end of the third trimester, when things have kicked into high gear. The baby shower is the perfect excuse to gather your loved ones and properly set the intention of joy, gratitude, celebration, and a positive vibration for you and the baby. It was important for me to be able to celebrate the birth of my daughter with a serious bang; so instead of one baby shower, I decided to split up the festivities into three different ones—one for the Latino contingency, one for the American gals, and one hosted by my gay friends aptly titled the "gaybe shower"—all of them excellent excuses to gather and rejoice in the most exciting time of my life.

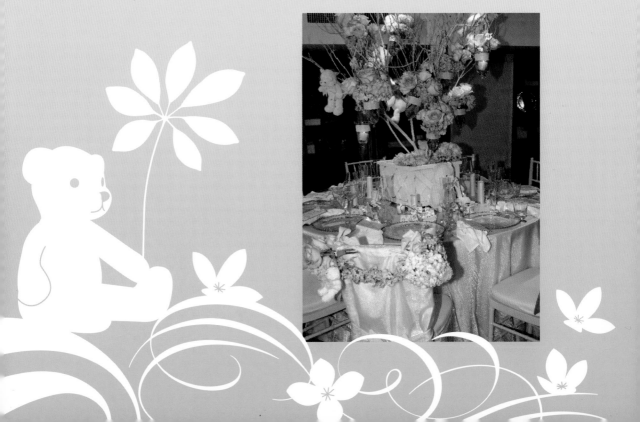

At the fiesta Mexicana, everything was pink and white, we sang karaoke, I lavished the place with chocolate fountains and massive bursts of rose bouquets, and I provided little trinkets, like barrettes and scarves, to my guests as party favors. For the American baby shower, I chose a slick, chic, Park Avenue–type affair, replete with pink champagne and a bountiful dessert table. For the infamous gaybe shower, I went for a more whimsical theme, which included playful lollipops and lively, colorful decor.

I'm not implying that everyone needs to throw three separate baby showers— I myself did it for purely logistical reasons. But what I am suggesting is that you open your mind, get creative, let loose, and have fun with the prospect of such a momentous celebration.

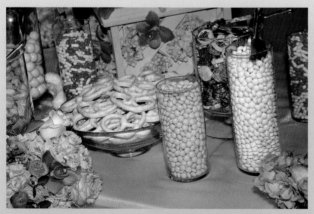
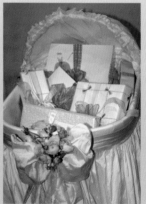
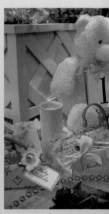

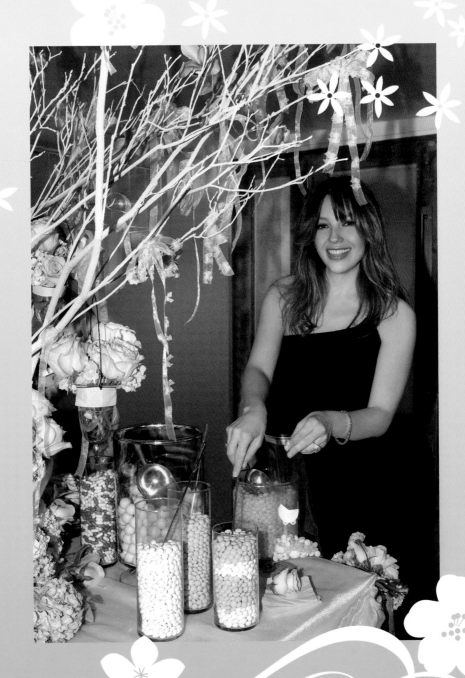

the labor lowdown

I imagine that all first-time mothers, like myself, probably spend the first eight months of their terms wondering endlessly how they will know when it is time, but then all of a sudden, when everything starts to shift inside (see "Heads Up: The Signs," page 125), you just know in your gut (literally) that it's all begun in earnest. But it does help to know ahead of time what each stage of labor will generally be like. Granted, since each woman will have her own thoughts and approach to how she will give birth (hospital delivery versus home birth, C-section versus vaginal, and so on), each woman's labor runs its course differently. Still, a few basics apply.

when to head to the hospital

I wish there were an absolute answer to the age-old question of when to go to the hospital or birthing center, but given the individual character of each pregnancy, and what each woman will prefer for her own experience, the answer each time will be completely different.

I wanted to be in the comfort and peace of my own home for as long as possible, enduring the bulk of the labor, intense as it was, in a more private and personal way. I knew that pre-labor, and even the beginning of real labor, could last for days, and I wanted to avoid the feeling of being one more woman on the maternity assembly line in the hospital and instead experience the entirety of the birth of my daughter in the most intimate manner possible, surrounded by calm and familiarity.

Typically, women are advised to call the midwife or doctor when contractions are between five and ten minutes apart. Effective contractions usually last 45 seconds to one minute in duration and are generally strong at the peak. Patience will be among your most important tools as you ride out the sometimes-lengthy labor. Get in touch with your team players—they will be able to assess your situation and know when it is time for you to head out.

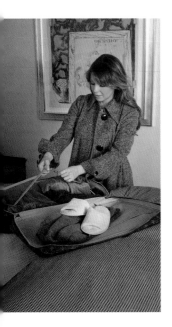

the stages of labor

The whole labor and delivery process averages fourteen hours for first-time mothers, so the first thing to accept is that labor is a *process*. There is no getting around the fact that in its natural state it takes its time. Since some preliminary contractions have started happening even in the second trimester, you will want to know how to differentiate them from the actual labor contractions as you get closer.

In the earliest stages of labor, some women have mild contractions for days at a time before the cervix even starts to budge, and they can last anywhere from thirty to forty-five seconds, recurring every five to thirty minutes. In other women, the cervix may efface (or thin out) and dilate a lot slower or a lot faster. Some of the symptoms at this time might include nausea, gastrointestinal distress, or back pain.

Actual labor contractions will start to last from a little over half a minute to about one minute, and will persist even after sips of water; in fact, they will become more frequent and stronger, occurring every three to five minutes, and might start more from the back area and move toward the front. You may feel sick to your stomach, experience incredible pressure, or have pain in your legs. By the time you are going through what is known as "active labor" you will hopefully be between four to seven centimeters dilated. Your contractions should be regular and persistent, occurring every three to five minutes, and lasting about a minute or so each. Most women are in "hard" or more accurately "active" labor way before they are ten centimeters dilated. Again, remember that these are just general numbers and can vary tremendously given individual circumstances.

During the second stage of labor (when you'll you be glad that you did your Kegel exercises), after your cervix is fully dilated, the contractions will remain at around sixty seconds usually recurring every three to five minutes. This stage could last anywhere from twenty minutes to several hours, until the baby is born, which may cause intense sensations of pressure and pain around the vagina and rectum. You may develop the sensation of having to go to the bathroom (to have a bowel movement) as the baby's head moves down the birth canal and presses on the rectum. Needless to say, the pain sensations will all vary greatly, depending on how much (if any) epidural is used (more on drugs later), and how much preparation—mental and physical—a woman has done in advance.

In the third and final stage of labor, the placenta or afterbirth is delivered, usually within twenty minutes of the baby's birth.

Okay . . . on paper, or maybe in biology class, all of this makes perfect sense, but when you're the one actually going through it, your levelheaded mind is not in charge. You may feel irrational anxiety or be seized by uncontrollable excitement. For this reason, during the labor you have to keep reminding yourself that all of the meditating and visualizations, all the prenatal yoga, and all the Kegel exercises you have done up to this point have been preparing you for perhaps the most challenging, but certainly the most special, moment of your life.

Drawing on the calmness of breath awareness and keeping a quiet focus, you will find that you are able to navigate the labor with natural fortitude. Other pain-management techniques include massage (by your doula or partner if he or she has been taking birthing courses with you) and taking a warm shower, as this can help relax and loosen the muscles. Mood music and aromatherapy, too, can certainly help bring you deep into relaxation; and the use of props like the birthing ball can also provide support, and perhaps some relief, during labor. For every pang of pain or every fear of uncertainty, try to use all your mental awareness to reverse the negative sentiment and instead focus on the miracle of creation and how amazingly lucky you are to be its divine vessel.

intentions versus interventions

Because each of us has such a unique set of circumstances, and each of our pregnancies plays out so differently, we have to mentally brace ourselves from the get-go for a Plan B that may have to kick in. For some women this may mean having to reluctantly agree to a C-section, and for others it may mean more drugs. Every "solution" comes with its own pros and cons, potential risks to the mother and/or baby, and, if things ever veer off track, doctors and midwives must take action accordingly. It can seem like every choice or option you encounter along the way turns out to be a calculated risk—it's one thing when you're three months pregnant and debating diagnostic screening tests with a girlfriend on your living room sofa. It's another thing entirely when you're on your back in a birthing bed, with your heart in your throat and your baby poised to make its move; you are not necessarily going to be in the best mental framework to assess important decisions. Staying informed ahead of time at least gives you the information you need so that if you do have to make a call, you can feel empowered to be your own advocate.

When people talk about *interventions* in the birthing world, they are referring to procedures undertaken to help your labor progress. Some doctors would argue that many of these so-called interventions are critical, while those from the natural birthing school of thought maintain that these interventions are totally unnecessary and perhaps even hazardous to the mother and child. Knowing what each of them entails will, at the very least, arm you with the knowledge to make an informed choice. Also, having a health-care provider (midwife or doctor) whom you are confident is your advocate will help to reduce confusion and eliminate doubt when these situations arise and interventions are advised or suggested.

fetal monitoring

Unless yours is considered a high-risk pregnancy or you have been given an epidural (which we'll talk about more in a moment) chances are you will not require electronic fetal monitoring. In the event that you do, there are two kinds of monitoring: the more common external monitoring, whereby a device is strapped to your belly to pick up the baby's heartbeat; or, when more precise results are needed, internal monitoring, which uses an electrode attached through your dilated cervix to the baby's scalp, allowing doctors to read the fetal heartbeat directly.

But today, for the low-risk mother, doctors and midwives typically feel that intermittent fetal heart checks are adequate. Research has shown that continuous electronic monitoring is no more efficient than manual fetal heartbeat checks every fifteen minutes or so, and every five minutes during the delivery itself. If you want to walk during your labor, this type of monitoring is fine. However if you plan to spend most of your labor in your birthing bed (especially if you've decided on an epidural), why not listen to the baby's heartbeat more continuously since there is no downside to knowing that the heartbeat is stable and reassuring.

forceps and vacuum extraction

When a baby seems to be having trouble getting through the birth canal, a doctor may decide that the delivery will require some assistance and opt to use forceps, a tool to carefully hold the baby's head and help it out. Alternatively, the doctor may use vacuum extraction, a suction device that attaches to the baby's head and gently pulls her out. Both practices, though quite useful and even necessary sometimes, can cause injury to both the mother and baby, so it is important that whoever is doing the procedure has solid experience with this kind of delivery. It is a good idea to discuss these alternative methods of delivery with your doctor ahead of time to make sure you are comfortable with their use during your delivery. They are important tools, occasionally necessary, usually used safely, and can help you avoid a C-section.

the episiotomy

The episiotomy (or "the dreaded snip," as I prefer to call it) is a small incision made in the perineum, the area between the anus and vagina, to enlarge the birth opening and help the delivery along. There are different schools of thought about whether it is beneficial or not. One believes that a clean surgical cut is conducive to an easier healing process, as otherwise the area may suffer a jagged tear requiring more stitches than would an episiotomy; the other school believes that if the skin is prepared properly, you will not need an episiotomy. These preparatory steps include massaging the perineum with oil regularly during the last three months of the term. Talk to your doctor or midwife about what else you can do to prepare this delicate piece of skin for the birth. Like other interventions, the procedure may be deemed necessary and can only really be assessed on a case-by-case basis. The American College of Obstetricians and Gynecologists maintains that episiotomies should be a last resort and not just a way to speed things up. Keep reminding yourself (and your team, if you feel pressured to decide) that labor is a process and that you are entitled to take your time.

the drugs debate

For most women, pain becomes redefined in the intensity of labor. For some of us, the physical pain can be extreme enough to warrant what is known as an epidural, the anesthesia most commonly used during labor, which blocks the nerves to the lower body but allows the mother to be alert through the process to experience the labor. Alternatively, some might argue that the epidural limits the complete holistic experience that a mother can feel.

Some women have found that having less pain helped them to relax and rest so that pushing during the second stage of labor was easier. This allowed them to experience their births with greater comfort and joy, rather than just the trauma of pain. However, it is important to know that there can be some undesirable side effects from an epidural. These can include severe migraine-like headaches, nausea, vomiting, and extreme itchiness. Some women also feel much more vulnerable and incapacitated if they become numb from the waist down. The good news is that epidural dosing can be adjusted so that this is not likely to happen. Advances in the types and doses of medication used for epidurals have allowed patients to be relieved of pain while minimizing the temporary paralysis (or inability to move one's legs) that used to occur. In fact, there is now something known as a walking epidural, which shows just how little interference with motor function there can be.

Something I was not prepared for was that after the baby is out and emotions are flying and everything is magical, after you're holding your baby, and even after you have cut the cord . . . the doctor still has the task of delivering the placenta from inside you and repairing your vagina if you had an episiotomy or sustained a tear. Usually, the placenta spontaneously separates from the uterus within a few minutes after the baby is born, and with gentle traction applied to the remaining portion of the umbilical cord it should come out easily and uneventfully. Although it can take up to two hours for the placenta to separate from the uterus, it typically separates within a few minutes after the delivery of the baby. After the obstetrician or midwife sees signs that the placenta has spontaneously separated from the uterus (a gush of blood, lengthening of the cord, and the uterus becoming globular) he or she will then apply gentle traction on the cord while asking the patient to give a little push. In rare circumstances when the placenta is abnormally adherent to the uterus and does not separate spontaneously, it is manually removed, which means a hand is inserted into the uterus and manually separates the placenta from the uterine wall.

I never imagined that I would get an epidural, certain that I had a high threshold for pain. But by the twenty-eighth hour of my labor, that epidural felt to me like the great mother of all martinis, a magical elixir of the gods, and the moment the anesthesiologist administered the drug was the moment my love affair with this gentle bald man began. He became my angel. The truth is that with the epidural, I felt like I could finally get through the rest of the labor . . . so much for going natural. The lesson here, ladies, is that you will simply have to have an open mind about things that may change within your plan, as you will find yourself having to make (and remake) decisions with every twist and turn that may come.

THE ORGAN RESHUFFLE

The first attempt at getting out of bed immediately following the delivery is going to feel strange, let me tell you. You will literally feel all of your intestines almost swoop back into place. During pregnancy, our inner organs and intestines rearrange themselves to make room for the growing baby. So when you get up from the bed for the first time after you've delivered, be prepared for the sensation of your organs seeming to slide back in place, each one somehow knowing exactly where to go.

to induce or not to induce

Inducing labor is another dicey topic, and the decision to do so depends on many variables, the most critical being the possibility of risk to the mother or baby. If there are no other presenting complications, doctors or midwives might want to induce labor because a woman is overdue (ten to fourteen days after your due date) or if her water breaks but her labor does not begin spontaneously after twenty-four hours have passed since the water broke.

Natural induction techniques include nipple stimulation, which releases the labor hormone oxytocin, and sexual intercourse, which has also been said to stimulate uterine contraction. Other methods include acupressure or acupuncture, or even just moving your body around a bit.

Medical induction is typically achieved through a synthetic hormone called pitocin, which stimulates the labor. Discuss the details and ramifications of this approach well in advance with your doctor or midwife so that you are not led to believe at the last minute when you are most vulnerable that a forced induction is the only way through your delivery. This hormone, though understandably necessary in certain scenarios and usually safe and effective, can stimulate contractions with an intensity that can sometimes cause the baby to go into distress (see "The C-section Question," on the facing page). A C-section might be fine for some women, but if you (like me) are intent on having a vaginal birth, and healthy enough to do so, you should be well informed about the possible effects of pitocin and how it can radically change the course of your experience. It is also important to keep in mind that pitocin is usually used safely and effectively and can help patients progress in their labors if they have been stalled or are not progressing properly.

Try to remember, no matter how raw you may feel in a moment of discomfort or fear, you still have to be your own advocate (or have your doula or partner speak for you if you have discussed your birthing plan ahead of time and you find that you are too incapacitated to speak for yourself).

Another method that a doctor or midwife might employ to help the labor along is to sweep or rupture the membranes, which stimulates the labor by helping to release prostaglandin (a hormone-like substance) from the amniotic sac into the mother's blood-stream. Cervical ripeners in the forms of vaginal gels or tablets may also be used by a doctor or midwife.

the c-section question

Given the rise of C-sections in the United States (the government announced an all-time high in 2006, after a 50 percent increase since 1996), it seems many have lost sight of the fact that labor is a natural process that is *supposed to last long*.

Maybe because C-sections are seen as "practical" when birth is looked at from a time- and pain-management standpoint, people (new moms and doctors alike) have distanced themselves from the natural expression and evolution of birth and, in doing so, possibly cheated the mothers out of the most amazing phenomenon in the world. These "designer deliveries" are not only more expensive and more invasive but can unnecessarily compromise a mother's chance to naturally participate in her experience.

But that is not to say that C-sections do not have their very important place in obstetrics. In fact, we all know that sometimes C-section deliveries are the only way to save lives, and obviously, in those instances, we should be grateful that medicine is advanced enough to be able to step in that way when complications do arise.

IT'S CALLED "LABOR" FOR A REASON

Like everything else in life, birthing comes with all kinds of risks and potential complications. But challenging as they may seem, we should acknowledge the far-reaching advances in medicine that have made almost every one of these impediments in some way manageable. Obviously, sometimes things are beyond anyone's control, but there is something that can be done to remedy most problems that arise during labor and birth. Think positively, and do not let this (or any other) book scare you into what I call "maternal hypochondria."

BREECH BABIES Most babies end up head downward in what is known as a vertex position. A breech presentation occurs when the baby's head is positioned upward, in either a footling breech, where the baby's foot (or feet) are pointing downward, or a traverse position, where the baby lies sideways and the buttocks face downward. In either case, these babies are rarely born vaginally. In fact, the American College of Obstetricians and Gynecologists strongly suggests C-section births for breech babies. Some doctors, midwives, and even acupuncturists are trained to help turn the baby head-down before the birth, either by physically manipulating the position from outside (called external cephalic version, or ECV) or through an ancient Chinese method known as moxibustion, which involves burning an herb called mugwort near a specific trigger point on the mother's foot.

PREECLAMPSIA Most prevalent in first-time pregnancies, typically after the seventh month, a condition known as preeclampsia (also known as toxemia, pregnancy-induced hypertension, or PIH) may arise. It affects 5 to 8 percent of all pregnancies and is characterized by high blood pressure and elevated levels of protein in the urine. Though it is highly treatable, if preeclampsia is not taken care of, it can lead to more serious problems for the mother and baby. Hamolysis Elevated Liver Low Blood Levels of Platelets (HELLP) syndrome is a more severe form of preeclampsia and should be diagnosed and treated by a doctor right away.

PROBLEMS WITH THE PLACENTA This happens when the placenta implants (attaches) to the lowermost portions of the uterus and blocks part or all of the cervix. Placenta previa is often detected by routine ultrasound at twenty weeks or earlier, and should also be suspected if you notice painless bright red vaginal bleeding particularly in the second and third trimesters. Placenta previa is a serious condition and usually necessitates early delivery (thirty-six to thirty-seven weeks) and usually by C-section.

Placenta accreta: When the placenta attaches too deeply into the uterine wall, it usually requires surgery to remedy. In severe cases of placenta accreta, unfortunately, a hysterectomy might be necessary.

Placental abruption: In this very serious complication, part or all of the placenta separates from the uterine wall before the birth of the baby. The baby, of course, cannot survive without blood from the placenta, and the mother can hemorrhage from the condition. Placental abruption may be detected through ultrasound, but there are also red-flag symptoms such as heavy vaginal bleeding or painful frequent contractions. Your doctor may recommend immediate delivery, possibly by C-section.

PRETERM LABOR When a baby is born before thirty-seven weeks in the womb, it is considered to be premature, or preterm, and this occurs in about 12 percent of births in the United States. The cause of preterm labor is unclear, though we do know that the earlier a baby is born before her due date, the more she is at risk for possible health complications. Most premature births will happen between weeks twenty-eight and thirty-seven, although babies have been able to survive being born as early as twenty-four weeks of gestation. Consult your doctor or midwife to see if you are at risk for preterm labor, discussing things like your age, your history of miscarriage (if applicable), your prenatal care regimen or any problems you may have had with your uterus. Signs of preterm labor might include cramping; diarrhea and/or frequent urinating; pressure in the back, pelvis, or abdomen; mucus-like bloody discharge; or rhythmic, persistent contractions that occur every ten minutes. If you have more than six contractions in one hour, you should call your doctor or midwife.

MULTIPLES Twin-to-twin transfusion syndrome (TTTS): This condition occurs when there is an uneven distribution of blood flow between twins sharing the same placenta. There are in-utero treatments to manage this through laser surgery or amniocentesis, but sometimes premature delivery may be necessary.

Vanishing twin syndrome: This condition, which affects 21 to 30 percent of multiple pregnancies, occurs when more than one fetus is seen during an early ultrasound, but in a later screening, only one is detected, and the pregnancy proceeds as a single pregnancy. The vanishing twin usually does not negatively affect the well-being of the remaining viable pregnancy.

THYROID IMBALANCE About one in two hundred pregnant women has hyperthyroidism, a condition in which the thyroid gland produces too much thyroid hormone. Those with too few hormones (hypothyroidism) may have difficulty conceiving, but if they do happen to get pregnant, they can be treated with additional hormone supplements to prevent miscarriage or other complications. Babies born to women with this condition usually have a low birth weight.

WEAKENED CERVIX A woman's cervix is weakened either from prior operations (such as cone biopsies, multiple dilation and curettage procedures and in particular, second trimester abortions) or from exposure in utero to medications such as DES. This condition is known as Cervical Incompetence. In this situation, the cervix cannot support the weight and strain of the growing fetus and the result is painless unsuspecting premature dilation of the cervix without contractions resulting in a second-trimester miscarriage in which the water suddenly breaks and a premature fetus is expelled. Cervical Incompetence can be treated with a procedure known as a cerclage, which uses a special stitch to help close and strengthen the cervix. The tricky part about this one is that the condition is often not diagnosed until after a second trimester miscarriage. Women who are felt to be at risk for Cervical Incompetence (patients with prior cervical operations or a history of DES exposure) can be followed closely with ultrasounds to measure cervical length and dilation. If cervical shortening or early dilation is detected, a cerclage can hopefully be placed emergently so as to prevent a miscarriage.

LOW BIRTH WEIGHT When a baby is born at less than 5 pounds, 8 ounces, he's considered to be at a low birth weight (also known as growth-restricted) and will likely need special medical attention and more time in the hospital. Premature babies and multiples are typically born underweight, although babies born at full term can also have a low birth weight.

STILLBIRTH In about one in two hundred pregnancies, fetal death, known as "stillbirth," will occur after week 20. There are many possible reasons, including umbilical cord problems, genetic abnormalities, infections, and placenta problems. Most stillbirths happen before labor has even begun.

the moment of truth

Just when the intensity of labor starts to reach the boiling point, and you feel like throttling that sweet nurse who's been telling you to take deep breaths, something miraculous starts to happen, the "something" that pretty much got you here in the first place: *LOVE*. Somehow, as your baby makes her way out, through the pain and sweat and raw force of all that's happening physiologically, from somewhere deep inside of you, there comes a surge of tenderness that just takes over and for a moment makes you the strongest woman in the world.

And before you know it, your little creature comes out crying at the top of her tiny little lungs, experiencing the first sensations of her new life: the warmth of your body, the rhythm of your heartbeat, and the smell of your skin. It is truly nature at its best, reminding womankind time and again that the term Mother Nature is not just a random choice of words. It is such a unique experience, like meeting a part of yourself for the first time.

I remember the precise moment when I saw her see me, our eyes locking for a split second, and in that moment both of us quietly realized that we had known each other all along. It just does not get any better than this.

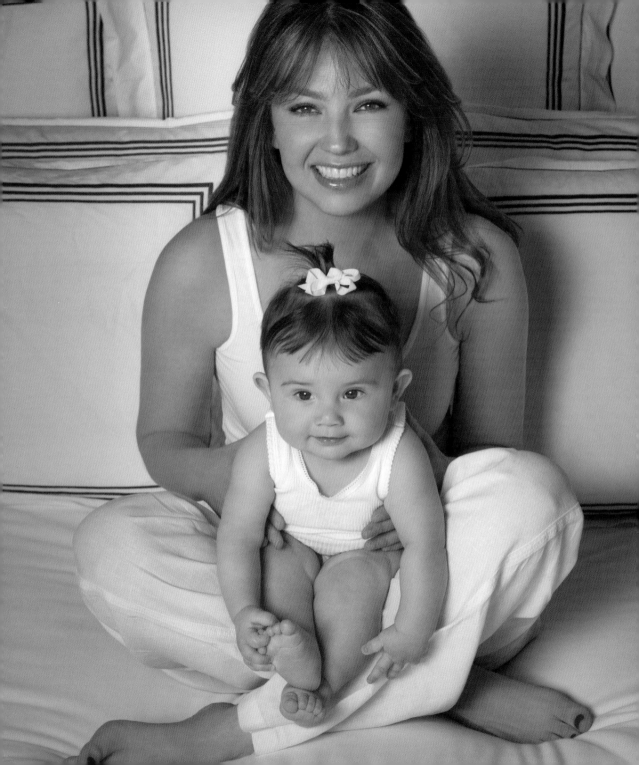

chapter 4: your brave new world
FOURTH TRIMESTER: POSTPARTUM

I didn't know that there was such a thing as a fourth trimester until I happened upon a DVD called *The Happiest Baby on the Block,* in which a doctor makes the point that even after a baby is born it is in many ways still a fetus. Your child, though now separate and outside of you, still implicitly relates to and is calmed by the scent, sound, and sight of you. Think of this period as a kind of primal sensory survival state, where it is *your* very presence that becomes the key to your baby's ultimate wellness and peace of mind.

Knowing this, we as mothers want to be nothing short of perfect for our newborns. For me, this notion became the crux of my postpartum intentions; however, I learned quickly that the raw reality of this delicate time is not exactly conducive to perfection, given the new adjustments that we must contend with. During the first few postpartum weeks I operated in a dream state, with emotions ranging from extreme joy to total shock, with a whole lot of confusion and uncertainty in between.

To gracefully endure these monumental changes and hold on to some semblance of peace and tranquility—for your own sake and the baby's—it is my belief that the most fundamental fourth-trimester coping tool is *patience*. In much the same way that you may have spent the first few months of your pregnancy adapting to life with a baby within, the first few months *after* the birth are also a time of transition, not to mention serious physical (and oftentimes emotional) recovery.

That said, if you are typically the kind of person who is hard on yourself, this is the time to *really* take it easy and cut yourself some slack. Coddle yourself, rest yourself, and try with all your might to love yourself, even if you don't love how you feel or what you look like in the mirror. Remember that, much like every other part of the pregnancy, this one, too, is temporary and fraught with surprises. The two critical parts of the fourth trimester are getting accustomed to your new life with a baby and getting back to your old self.

This chapter covers some of the various physical and medical issues that will come up, for both you and the baby, and explores the various, oftentimes confusing facets of the new mental landscape of motherhood. We also discuss nutrition and exercise and how to tackle the ever-pressing issues of weight loss and beauty, the two seemingly insurmountable hurdles (key word: *seemingly*) that arise postpartum.

Above all, as you face your own postpartum period, no matter how volatile or uncomfortable you may feel, by understanding that pregnancy has a beginning, middle, and end, you can see a finish line, where distress ends and family begins.

dealing with discomforts … and the many untold truths within the secret society

Two weeks before my due date, one of my closest friends came to visit, and in her hand was a mysterious little bag. Curious, I asked her what it was. "Open it later and call me," she replied. Inside the bag I found small, peculiar-looking squirt bottles, witch hazel pads, maxi pads large enough for the crotch of Godzilla, and a few sets of disposable hospital underwear.

When I looked inside this little bag I almost fainted, because up to that moment, all I had heard from everyone were lighthearted pep talks and pink balloons. No one talks about the *real* tribulations of postpartum care to a first-time mom who's already on edge about everything else that a pregnancy entails. Our loved ones and even our closest friends protect us from the not-so-pleasantries, sparing us the details and allowing us to get there on our own. My aforementioned friend was the one who gave it to me straight, so let me be the one to give it to you straight right here.

Let's not kid ourselves: The postpartum period can be as challenging as those first few months when you were vomiting your way through the day, your body adjusting to its new cocktail of hormones and your belly slowly taking charge of your life. But the aftermath of birth brings with it an entirely *new slew* of physical challenges, as your organs shift back into place and the body recovers from the process of labor. Your breasts will become the two great planets around which all of life will seem to orbit, and you may feel more tired and physically drained than you could have ever imagined possible.

The truth is that it will be different for every woman, depending on what kind of birth took place: Mothers who had C-sections and episiotomies, for example, have essentially endured delicate surgeries, which require time and plenty of rest until the healing is complete. Though each mother's process of restoration will be unique, given how complicated or straightforward her own delivery may have been, or what kind of personality the baby has, the key to getting through the postpartum time is to honor this final frontier of pregnancy. Acknowledge that the fourth trimester is a natural and necessary part of the healing experience for both mother and baby, because the two of you went through a shock in birth. Whatever comes up, do not be afraid; you've been through the worst of it, and by now you are a seasoned pro in the art of endurance.

tips

Familiarize yourself with this general list of symptoms and conditions that may arise as your body heals. This way, you'll have fewer surprises and more time to recover.

❋ **Abdominal pain or cramping:** Not unlike mild contractions or menstrual discomfort, these pains occur as the uterus contracts back to its original size during a process known as involution, which can take anywhere from four to six weeks. Ways to avoid and sometimes treat abdominal pain include not sitting or standing with your legs crossed, drinking plenty of water, stretching your muscles regularly, and taking little walks.

❋ **Baby blues:** Not to be confused with postpartum depression (see "Gentle on the Mental," page 178), which is a lot more serious, baby blues can kick in, lasting for a few days or a few weeks, during which time you experience moodiness or even some sadness. Book yourself a day at the spa and get yourself nice and pampered, which is something that always cheers me up. Talking about your feelings with your partner, friends, or family is also therapeutic and healthy for the psyche.

❋ **Bleeding:** Heavy, bloody vaginal discharge will occur for about a month to six weeks after the birth, as all of the remaining tissues and fluids are released from the uterus. The blood is bright red and typically appears as thick clots or mucus in the beginning, lightening up to brownish or yellow spotting as it subsides. Use supersize sanitary napkins or disposable underwear for the first few weeks, but do not use tampons for at least six weeks after delivery. But perhaps worse than the sight of all that raw blood is the smell it brings with it. I made sure to keep aromatic candles and oils like lavender and eucalyptus in my bathroom and in the common areas where I'd host visitors. (Note: These scents may be too strong for the baby's room.) If you feel that bleeding has gone on too long (past a month), consult your doctor.

✳ **Bloodshot eyes:** Red eyes and/or dark circles around the eyes can result from pushing during delivery. Chilled slices of cucumber on the eyes are refreshing and help to brighten the eyes.

✳ **Breast problems:** Cracked nipples or engorgement due to breastfeeding may occur. See "Breast Intentions," page 170, for ways to get your girls feeling better.

✳ **C-section scar:** Women who have undergone C-sections will also have a post-op incision to contend with; after a few days it will tighten and seal. Over time, the scar should start to fade, and vitamin E can be used to further lighten the mark. Contact your doctor if you suspect an infection in the area or if the scar feels painful beneath the surface.

✳ **Epidural side effects:** Epidurals can sometimes leave some residual symptoms that include nausea, headaches, itching, leg numbness, and soreness at the site of the injection. Anesthesia can also cause constipation, which you can relieve with a stool softener, enema, or suppository. For the itching, try applying some chamomile lotion, and if the nausea gets really bad, consult with your doctor about other possible treatments.

✳ **Exhaustion:** No getting around this one, it just comes with the territory. You can try to get ahead of the exhaustion by making sure you are getting seven to eight hours of sleep nightly, which I know is easier said than done. See "Counting Sheep, Yearn to Sleep," page 180, for tips on catching your Zs.

❊ **Gas and bloating:** Slow digestion and trapped air in the belly can cause severe gas and bloating, easily treatable with enemas and suppositories.

❊ **Hair loss:** Some women experience extreme hair loss after giving birth, a condition known as postpartum alopecia. Generally, hair will start to grow back within the next year and a half, and depending on how noticeable it is on you, experimenting with new styles can help to ease the transition.

❊ **Hemorrhoids and fissures:** It's possible to get these grapes of wrath from pushing during labor and delivery, as well as fissures, which are tiny tears in the skin around the anus. Sometimes the hemorrhoids are minor—but other times these little monsters explode from within the anus like some sort of unruly, purposefully destructive force, leaving one's bottom unmercifully raw. There are excellent hemorrhoid-relieving creams, such as the old faithful Preparation H, to relieve the irritation and quell the burn, and a stool softener also helps things along so that you don't have to work so hard. There is also a fabulous little invention that might just be as relieving to an overly irritated bum as it is embarrassing to lug around—the notorious *donut*. The donut is a pillow-like tube-shaped mobile seat you can take anywhere, making the prospect of sitting viable.

❊ **Incontinence and difficulty going to the bathroom:** The first poop is another subject no one is dying to discuss. Women are scared to push, and everything stings. Thankfully one of my sisters filled me in on how to prepare for this dilemma by instructing me to eat lots of fiber and drink tons of prune juice as I got close to delivery; she also insisted I start taking a stool softener immediately after the birth. . . . Never mind the notion of wiping afterward, especially if you have stitches on your perineal area like a bridge from Manhattan to New Jersey. I quickly learned what the squirt bottles and witch hazel pads from my friend's goodie bag were for!

Some women also experience postpartum incontinence (leaking urine), because the pelvic floor is weakened after the birth, and most women find themselves urinating more often than normal as the body gradually releases all of the water that accumulated during the pregnancy. If incontinence is a problem, don't be afraid to wear adult undergarments like Depends, and know that this too shall pass.

❋ **Night sweats:** The hormonal changes that occur after you give birth can cause any number of different problems, one being night sweats. I had to sleep with three to four sets of pajamas and underwear next to my bed, because I would wake up soaked in my own sweat, leaving puddles of perspiration on every square inch of my sheets. To aid your body in eliminating the hormones you no longer need, drink plenty of water throughout the day, and at night put a towel under your sheets to soak up excess sweat.

❋ **Sleep issues:** For so many reasons, both logistical and physiological, women will suffer from sleep deprivation during their pregnancy, and certainly after they give birth. If it is a case of restlessness or insomnia, a bit of exercise each day can help, as can a soak in a warm tub before bed. Unfortunately, getting up in the middle of the night to tend to a crying or hungry baby is simply unavoidable.

❋ **Soreness of the perineum:** General soreness and stinging of the vagina and/or perineum is common. If your nether-petals hadn't swollen during pregnancy, they will swell and very likely hurt like hell for several days after the delivery. The vagina, tough as she is to be able to endure the miracle of birth, also happens to be one of the most delicate parts of your body. The poor thing will sting, burn, itch, and irritate. To tame the flame, try sitting on an ice pack; not only does it cool your business, but it's also generally invigorating when you're not feeling tip-top. You can also dab the area with witch hazel pads, or consider sitting in a cool sitz bath, which is a traditional European method of soaking just the hips and buttocks, typically to relieve any discomforts related to the pelvic area. You can find plastic sitz baths at most drug stores and pharmacies.

baby wellness

Just as your body evolves through its own process of recalibration, your baby will also undergo some temporary physical conditions post-birth that you should be aware of, so you don't automatically freak out if, say, your baby looks more like a tiny old man to you than the angelic newborn child you had envisioned.

Babies are sometimes born with subtle red markings on some parts of their bodies known as "stork bites," or even tiny pimples known as baby acne, or milia. Other babies get a rash called erythema toxicum that resembles mosquito bites, while some are born with actual patches of bluish or purple skin. Most babies come out covered in vernix, the oily white substance that protects their skin; some babies, especially premature ones, are also born with bits of lanugo, a soft, hair-like fuzz that eventually disappears.

Being pushed through the narrow birth canal sometimes causes a baby's facial features to look squashed, or the shape of the head to appear elongated in what is called a "conehead" shape. Sometimes babies are also born with swollen genitals or nipples as a result of the mother's hormones.

As unsettling as some of these may seem at first, try to think of them as divine quirks of birth, and know that ultimately they will all go away.

baby's first tests

Moments after your baby is born, and for the next few days, your doctor, midwife, or pediatrician will administer a series of preliminary tests and treatments to ensure that everything is running smoothly. These include:

❋ The Apgar test, performed at one and five minutes after birth, which evaluates the baby's reflexes, muscle tone, heart rate, skin color, and breathing

❋ Weighing and measuring length and head circumference

❋ Antibiotic eye drops applied as a precaution against certain infections

❋ A vitamin K injection to aid in blood clotting

❋ A thorough pediatric examination by either your own pediatrician (if he or she is affiliated with the hospital in which you gave birth) or the hospital's

❋ State-mandated screening tests, which vary

❋ An optional hepatitis B shot—discuss this with your pediatrician in advance

breast intentions

It is no secret that breast milk is the most optimal form of nutrition for a newborn baby, a natural superfood that is unique to each child. It not only quells your little one's first hunger pangs but also provides her with powerful building blocks for digestive and neurological development, as well as arming her with antibodies against infections of many kinds. Before the mature breast milk comes in after about five days, the mother will produce a substance called colostrum, which is translucent, low in fat, and packed with protein.

Breastfeeding also has advantages for the mom, providing (but not limited to) bone fortification, weight loss, lower risk of certain kinds of cancers, and aiding in the process of uterine shrinking. Let's not forget that breast milk will cost you nothing, economizing things a bit.

BOSOM BUDDIES

The physiology of every mother-baby combination is so individually nuanced that essentially there is no "right way" to breastfeed. The trick is to experiment with various positions to discover what works best for you. Like all new moms, you will likely be timid at first, not knowing exactly how to handle, or even hold, your baby during a feeding. In time, though, after a little practice and a sense of what feels right, you'll become a pro. Here are a few classic positioning ideas to get you started:

Basic cradle hold: This is the most common position, with baby cradled in the mother's arms, lying across her chest. Make sure the baby's neck doesn't twist; try to fully face him to your breast to allow for easier swallowing.

Football clutch: In this position, the baby lies against the side of the mother's body, beneath her arm, which helps to keep the baby in place. It also gives the mother a better view of the latch.

Lying down on your side: This is a great position if you are tired and want to rest while you feed, as it relieves you of having to prop the baby up, since you are both lying on the same surface. Only use this once you're comfortable latching the baby on.

Despite all of the benefits that breastfeeding can yield for all parties involved, the process is not always as straightforward as one might expect. Even the most gung-ho among us, those who have dreamed endlessly about the sacred suckling, are likely to encounter unexpected challenges like cracked nipples, tenderness, engorgement, or a combination of all of the above. Or maybe (if you're in my shoes) your baby simply doesn't *want* to latch on, because the lazy little thing doesn't want to have to work for it.

For me, it was very important to be able to breastfeed my daughter. I knew that the key to successful breastfeeding would be not only my willingness and strong desire to do it, but also my daughter's ability to properly latch on. I soon learned that getting more of my areola (not just the nipple!) in her mouth meant more effective milk flow from my breast. Friends were quick to inform me that tickling the baby's upper lip would help to get her mouth open as wide as possible, and the more confident my movements were, the less awkward the process felt. Even though my daughter and I were a team on this complex breastfeeding mission, I had to be the one to drive it. Any sense of shame, insecurity, or doubt would only get in my way of establishing what I knew would ultimately be one of the most physically and emotionally beneficial aspects of this ever-special connection.

engorgement

At one point, my breasts became so engorged and painful that even the lightest grazing of a sheet against my nipples would cause excruciating pain. I knew that I would have to find solutions quickly, not only because I wanted to breastfeed more than anything in the world, but also because I needed to be able to somehow manage the pain. I enlisted the support of a lactation consultant, who was not only able to help me but also quickly dispelled myths about how to handle breastfeeding complications.

Engorgement occurs when the breasts become filled with milk faster than they are being drained. This can cause massive, hardened, painful breasts that ache endlessly. I was always led to believe that warm compresses could alleviate this condition, under the assumption that the heat would help to dilate the milk ducts and ease the flow. However, the lactation consultant informed me that the opposite could occur: The heat, she explained, can increase blood flow to the area, causing swelling and making things worse. If the milk is not drained in a timely manner, it can lead to an infection of the breast.

To manage the pain, I was instructed to take an Advil every eight hours as needed (taking it too often can mask fever) and to massage the breasts while nursing in order to dissolve any hardened cyst-like formations. The lactation consultant advised me to locate the little masses with my fingers and, with small, precise, concerted motions, to use the tips of my fingers to push on them, to actually try to squeeze them out, following them with my fingertips from the base of the breast toward the nipple until I felt them lessen and soften. I was also put on a routine of pumping every three hours to relieve the engorgement, so I ended up freezing a lot of my milk, which was also very handy. Believe me, a few weeks of pumping will give you a lot of storage. But pumping is only necessary when the baby cannot or is not available to remove the milk effectively.

Even more illuminating was the consultant's suggestion to place frozen green cabbage leaves and/or ice packs directly in the nursing bra around my breasts, leaving the nipples exposed, to relieve engorgement. I chose to wrap the leaves with clear plastic wrap to prevent them from leaking cold water on me. Bizarre as it sounds, it actually helped, and in no time I found myself looking into the eyes of my daughter as she drank my milk with perfect little rhythmic puckers of her tiny little mouth. This to me was ultimate nirvana.

feeding times

It is commonly said that breastfeeding often (eight to twelve times a day) is the best way to maximize nursing success, since it keeps the momentum of the milk flow active and continuous. The amount of milk a woman produces is directly related to the amount of milk her baby requires, so the more you feed, the more you'll refill with milk, and the less he feeds, the less milk your body will produce.

Learning your baby's hunger signs will also become crucial in knowing when it is time to feed. A fussy, crying baby is likely ready for his meal, as is a baby whose mouth puckers up. Watch your baby closely to learn his signals so that you can start to communicate early on about this delicate symbiotic process.

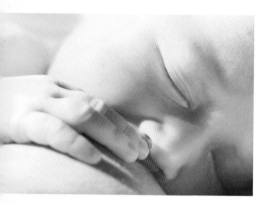

breast or bottle?

I decided that mixing breast and bottle would be the most reasonable way to ensure proper, hassle-free nutrition for my daughter. I quickly learned how to pump my own breast milk so that she would always have food on hand, whether I was able to feed her directly or not. There are many types of pumps out there—manual, electric, hospital grade, and even battery operated—and prices and user-friendliness vary. Consult your doctor or midwife and friends to get a sense of what might work best for you. If you decide to pump, which comes in handy if you are a busy mom, remember that all of the feeding gear needs to be thoroughly sterilized before the first use and must be kept meticulously clean by being thoroughly washed after each use.

A word of warning: For me, the first pump felt as if someone were tugging on my breasts, and instead of milk being extracted out, something seemed to be cutting me from the outside in. But this pain isn't experienced by everyone, and if it happens to you, know that it will subside. After you pump a few times you will get used to the sensation, your boobs will toughen up, and, as with everything else, you just learn to deal.

For some women, exclusive breastfeeding isn't an option for several reasons, be they schedule-driven, sexuality-driven, or simply (though nothing is ever simple) because the mother is not able to produce enough milk. For some women, the pain of breastfeeding is so unbearable that, despite all attempts to make it happen, the process is stripped of all joy and the bonding that is supposed to be happening instead instills a sense of dread. No mother or child should have to endure this. Breastfeeding should not be painful after the first week or so. If it is, contact a lactation consultant, midwife, doctor, or doula. With the proper help, you can likely soon experience painless breastfeeding.

If you are going the formula route, which is perfectly acceptable and may be convenient for all kinds of reasons (not the least of which is that your partner and other family members and friends can help with feedings), for the first twelve months of his life your baby should be drinking iron-fortified formula. Beyond that, the specific type of milk you choose will depend on your baby's needs. Some children, for example, are more sensitive to lactose, in which case, a soy-based formula might be ideal. Other babies will require even more specialized types, depending on other variables, such as allergies.

In the first six months, your baby should be eating at least every three to four hours. In time, you will start to recognize your baby's hunger patterns and needs. You should consult her pediatrician about quantities, as baby sizes vary, and so does the amount of milk they will each require. Newborns should be consuming at least 2 to 3 ounces every three or four hours; at one month old, they should go up to 4 ounces every four hours; and at six months, they should be drinking 6 to 8 ounces roughly every four or five hours during a twenty-four-hour period.

You'll want to look for Bisphenol A (BPA)–free feeding products. According to my daughter's pediatrician, glass bottles and the liners for drop-in bottles have never contained BPA. BPA is a plastics chemical and artificial estrogen currently used to manufacture polycarbonate plastics, like those used for most plastic baby bottles and other child-feeding products. BPA is also used to make epoxy linings of food cans, like those for infant formula, and other packaging, like the lids on jarred baby food.

In April 2008, the National Toxicology Program of the National Institutes of Health (NIH) determined that BPA poses risks to human development, linking exposure to it, even in small doses, to breast and prostate cancer as well as behavioral and reproductive problems.

Although the Food and Drug Administration (FDA) has yet to tighten safety standards, Wal-Mart, Toys "R" Us, and other retailers are removing BPA-containing products from store shelves. To find the BPA status of a particular brand of baby bottle, pacifier, teether, et cetera, consult the "Z Report on BPA in Children's Feeding Products" at http://zrecs.blogspot.com. The site also offers a text-messaging service to query the Z Report about a product's BPA content from your mobile phone.

Remember that each part of the bottle (the body, cap, and nipple) must be thoroughly sterilized before the first usage and after each usage thereafter. The easiest way to sterilize feeding equipment is to boil the gear in a pot for at least five minutes and let it air-dry on a clean towel.

Thankfully, there are many ways to bring proper nutrition to your baby, and while breast-feeding is miraculous at its best, it certainly isn't the only viable option. Consult your doctor, midwife, or doula to devise the best possible game plan for you and your little one. I found The Upper Breast Side (www.upperbreastside.com) in New York City, which was very helpful and informative. Also, The Pump Station is a great resource for any and all products for nursing mom and baby (www.pumpstation.com).

LACTATION STATION

Even though the act of breastfeeding seems like the most natural thing in the world, it can oftentimes be a very challenging process. We now have many modern tools to ease the way, however, and getting geared up early on is always a good idea. Here is a list of items that should be part of your personal lactation station. They don't need to go with you every-where, but having them on hand will make things a whole lot easier:

✳ Breastfeeding pillow

✳ Breast pads, as your nipples will inevitably leak

✳ Breast pump

✳ Burp cloths to wipe up any spit-up

✳ Comfortable rocking chair or glider in a calming area of your home

✳ Soothing nipple ointment to relieve cracking or irritation, such as olive oil or pure lanolin creams, which are safe for the baby and don't have to be washed off before nursing. Purelan and Lansinoh are companies that make excellent lanolin ointments, and both are available online. Pain or cracking which doesn't improve after the first week needs further evaluation.

✳ Supportive nursing bra

✳ And finally, stick to a balanced diet to ensure that you are getting a well-rounded dose of nutrients

gentle on the mental

Nothing will ever prepare you for the phenomenon of motherhood. It appears like some kind of celestial storm in your world, and aside from the unending love-flow that essentially defines life with a baby, having a child also provides us, as adults, with the unique opportunity to witness firsthand the miracle of watching a human develop from scratch. Consider it the science class of all science classes, only this time, you will play the part of both teacher and student, simultaneously educating yourself *and* learning from your own mistakes.

But along with the love and wonder and all the pastel fuzziness that your new world will entail, birth and babies can also inspire endless anxiety, confusion, paranoia, insecurity, and a whole slew of other negative mental states—which, by the way, are *all totally normal*, not only for physiological reasons (those dreaded hormones in flux again) but also because being a first-time mother is chock-full of emotional ramifications. That said, as you begin to care for this tiny new human in your life, and to keep as level a head as possible, it is imperative that you keep reminding yourself that *you are human*, too.

We have all heard about postpartum depression (PPD), but few of us realize that emotional imbalance after birth comes in all kinds of dimensions and levels of severity. You might be blissful now that your proverbial bundle of joy has arrived, or, if you are like me, you might find yourself missing your belly like an old friend whose presence you long for.

But for many women, postpartum depression is a condition that kicks in with a vengeance, giving rise to all kinds of deep, negative, and often long-lasting feelings of isolation, sadness, apathy, and lack of bonding with the baby. It is important to know that these psychological side effects of birth are common and nothing to be ashamed of.

There are two other forms of PPD that are prevalent: postpartum anxiety, in which mothers feel unnecessarily nervous around their baby and often don't leave the house for fear that something terrible might happen to them or the baby, and postpartum psychosis, whereby a mom will actually go into an alternate state of awareness, may have hallucinations, and may harm the baby. PPD isn't the "baby blues," which typically lasts from two days to two weeks; it is much more serious and requires prompt attention. Moms fearing they have PPD should seek help immediately, and with the support of family and professionals, it can be overcome.

While therapy and medication can certainly help in the more dire situations, I believe that true healing begins on the inside: Just as you learned how to face the demons while you were pregnant, you can also learn how to confront the emotional challenges now that you aren't. Like everything else, it starts with your will.

If yoga and meditation served you well during your term, it will likely continue to do so well after you've given birth. Understandably, physical and mental exhaustion may not be conducive to a complete wellness regimen, but the more you are able to practice silence and stillness, the closer you will get to a sense of equanimity in the face of the postpartum conundrum. Carving out time for yourself—be it for reading, cooking, knitting, catching up on e-mails, filing your nails, or any other activity that cools your jets—is critical for peace of mind, and the sooner you begin to do it after you have given birth, the sooner you will find peace. But if you find yourself at a total loss when it comes to personal spirit-lifting, here are some tips for inspiration that helped me:

Fuss management: Though the exact cause is unclear, many newborn babies suffer from colic, possibly attributable to the baby's individual temperament or some kind of gastrointestinal distress (though usually nothing to worry about medically). Babies with colic are usually more sensitive to things around them and may require a bit more atten-tion. Things you can try to relieve a colicky baby include: rocking her in your arms or in a cradle, rubbing her belly gently, wrapping her in a soft blanket, or taking her for a walk in the stroller or in the car for a drive (car seat a must!).

The unhelpful partner: If you find yourself juggling all of the feedings, chores, medical issues, and your own mental health at once, you might have an unhelpful partner on your hands. I believe the best antidote to this scenario is good old-fashioned communi-cation. Talk frankly, but diplomatically, with your partner about concerns and grievances, and together come up with a written plan for divvying up the duties. Certain things like breastfeeding will obviously be relegated to you as the mother, but your partner can certainly pitch in with groceries, cooking, bottle feedings, and household cleaning. Make a plan, and try to have fun with it.

Counting sheep, yearn to sleep: Not getting enough sleep is not only annoying but also extremely unhealthy. How can you be the best mommy in the world when all you can think about is curling up in the fetal position and dozing off? In addition to exercise and warm baths before bedtime, there is a fantastic yoga posture called the half-tortoise that is meant to help regulate the sleep-wake cycle. Sit on your knees, Japanese-style, with your torso straight. Raise both arms above your head, with both palms touching, and thumbs crossed. Take a deep breath, and with a straight spine, bend forward from your hips, keeping your core tight and your arms and elbows perfectly straight. Rest your forehead gently on the floor, making sure your chin doesn't tuck in toward your chest, with the tip of your nose just grazing the floor. Take ten deep breaths in this position.

educate while you regulate

Like most new moms, you will likely be spending quite a bit of time at home in the weeks after you give birth, recuperating, resting, and adjusting to a feeding schedule. Your baby, in the interim, will be doing a whole lot of sleeping, which will, in turn, afford *you* some quiet time. I found it extremely gratifying to use this downtime productively by reading books and articles about babies and parenting, and gradually getting myself into an informed mindset. The more I would read and digest, the less daunted and more confident I would feel as I continued to interact with my daughter. Reading, after all, is in many ways a type of focused meditation that lends itself to quiet, peacefulness, and, of course, innumerable insights.

partner praising

Sexual pleasure is an entirely personal experience: Some women might be counting the minutes until their next orgasm, but most will likely feel sexually off-limits for some time after the birth. Since parenting is a tag-team effort, though, your partner will also need some coddling as you both navigate this new chapter of the relationship. To that end, it is important to understand that sex is not the only way to establish intimacy and strengthen the bond, and there are other things you can do to experience profound connection with your mate.

After the reality of my husband seeing me through the volatile stages of pregnancy and birth—crying, feeling vulnerable, being hysterical, yelling at him, throwing things, going crazy, wearing no makeup, having dark circles under my eyes, and then actually watching close-up as I birthed our child, my legs wide open, my vagina in full dilation, blood dripping everywhere—I thought to myself, "How in God's name am I going to bring sexy back? How can I brainwash this man into forgetting what he saw, so that I can forever remain in his mind the beautiful angel of his life?"

So, one week after I gave birth, I decided to organize a surprise party for him, except the only guests would be the two of us. I had his secretary book his day full of appointments to keep him out of the house until late in the night. When he got home from work that evening, as he got out of the car, he could already hear the band that I had brought in to play live for us. The poor guy was baffled, yet through the window I could see the corners of his mouth gradually turning up into a smile.

I had (against all odds) managed to stuff myself into an industrial strength girdle, did full hair and makeup, and wore a stunning Ralph Lauren gown. I was fully bejeweled and perfumed, and the moment he walked into the house, with the straightest face possible, I quietly asked him, "Are you hungry, darling?" What followed was a full-scale production of a five-course meal, the most romantic, intimate, and cozy dinner we have ever shared, replete with music, wine, candlelight, fresh roses, delicious fare, and the best company ever—each other.

What can I say? This grown man *wept*. He kissed and hugged me, and said it was the most special night of his life, third only to our wedding and the birth of our daughter. The icing on the cake was when I cued the musicians to play the song that he sang to me at our wedding; as the song began, our newborn daughter was brought out so that the three of us could dance the song together. The guy went *nuts*.

So, the moral of the story is that sex is not everything. I knew that, somehow, I needed to give this man his woman back—and it worked. I understand that this is an over-the-top way of doing something special, but I guarantee that if you look inside, you, too, can find your own way. Consider hiring a babysitter (or square it away with your baby nurse or nanny in advance) and plan a surprise night out to dinner at your partner's favorite restaurant. You can do other types of things, like booking a couple's massage in your home, which can take place while the baby naps; or get tickets for a sporting event or performance that you know he or she will appreciate. Just make sure to carve out some time for your partner, a gesture that says, *thank you and I love you.*

still a table for two

With all of the anxiety I felt during those postpartum weeks, every night I would devour half of a pecan pie with half a pint of milk. I was eating emotionally and exhausted from breastfeeding, so I would just eat that pie as some kind of psycho-emotional redemption. Don't do what I did. Do not indulge with zero abandon—okay, maybe every three days you can eat a brownie if you must.

It really isn't rocket science: The more mindful you were regarding diet throughout your pregnancy, the easier it will be for you to shed the baby weight after the birth through diet and exercise. But even Jenny Craig herself wouldn't be able to snap right back into shape straight out of the delivery room, and realistically, most of us will be dealing with postpartum pounds for months to come. The good news is that breastfeeding is one of Mother Nature's most effective fat-shedding mechanisms, and the better news is that once you have really started to feel better, the prospect of exercise will stop being such a far-fetched notion.

Try not to fixate on losing weight by gently reminding yourself that for the first month or so after the birth you are still very much in recovery mode, and that you will require adequate nutrition, especially if you are breastfeeding. Breastfeeding organizations, such as La Leche League, say that less than 1,800 calories per day will negatively impact milk production—something to keep in mind as you design menus and meals. Likewise, when you are breastfeeding you should be conscious of your calcium intake, which is key for the baby's development and passes through the milk you produce.

Regardless, getting back into shape when you are no longer pregnant, in many ways, is no different than trying to *stay in shape* when you are: The key is to stick with fresh whole foods, drink lots of water, keep sugar intake low, and keep carbohydrates brown (brown rice, whole grain bread, whole wheat pasta, and so on). If you are breastfeeding, focus less on calorie-counting (since you'll need 500 to 600 *additional* calories for lactation) and more on consuming the right kinds of nutrient-rich foods. Make it a point to eat foods that are rich in calcium, like soymilk and kale, which is also rich in folate, another critical protein-building vitamin. Oranges and fresh orange juice are also high in folate. Foods rich in iron, like beans, lean red meat, and enriched breakfast cereals, should also be on your list, especially since you're likely to be losing a good amount of blood in the month after the delivery. Foods with fatty acids are also a critical part of the postpartum diet, so salmon, avocados, and nuts are great to keep in the regimen. And you'll get plenty of the necessary whole grains and fibers by eating brown rice, quinoa, millet, barley, and cooked oats.

Every breastfeeding mother should also consult her doctor, midwife, or pediatrician about what to avoid consuming. There are different stances on caffeine and alcohol consumption, for example, so checking with your support team is really the best way to get a handle on what is right for you.

Finally, just as your doctor suggested a prenatal supplement regimen for you at the start of your pregnancy, he or she should work with you to devise a postnatal supplement plan as well. Whatever is prescribed, make sure you stick to it diligently: You are still eating for two if you are a breastfeeding mother, and even if you're not, your body will need certain vitamins and minerals as it readjusts after delivery.

keep a postpartum metabolism in check

Here are five ways to maintain a steady and active metabolism. Follow these tips and you're sure to slim down at a healthy rate. Eat many small meals a day, instead of a few huge ones:

✳ Drink lots of water

✳ Plan for healthy, nutrient-rich snacks that you can have on the go or between baby chores

✳ Stay away from salty foods, or foods high in sugar or fat

✳ Make time to sit and eat slowly, as opposed to stuffing your face to save time

POSTPARTUM PROVISIONS

Here's a hit list of must-eats after the baby is born. Copy this and stick it on your fridge:

Fish: salmon, trout, cod

Meat: white-meat chicken, turkey, lean red meat

Nuts: pecans, almonds, cashews

Vegetables: kale, spinach, tomatoes, corn, potatoes, cauliflower, broccoli, peas

Fruits: strawberries, blueberries, pears, bananas, dried fruits

Grains: whole wheat bread, quinoa, brown rice, cream of rice, barley, cream of wheat, oatmeal

pour on the protein

These tried-and-true, protein-rich recipes are easy to follow and perfectly delicious. What's more, they'll not only save you time—they'll save you from your love handles as well!

TURKEY MEATBALLS

This is another favorite from Esther Blum, simple to make and perfect to freeze.

1 pound ground turkey breast

⅓ cup quick-cooking oats

½ cup grated Parmesan cheese

¼ teaspoon garlic powder

2 egg whites

Preheat the oven to 350°F. Spray a baking pan with nonstick cooking spray. In a medium bowl combine all the ingredients and shape into 1-inch balls. Place the meatballs in the baking pan. Bake for 20 minutes or until no longer pink. Remove from the pan and enjoy. You can also serve these with whole wheat pasta and a sauce made of sautéed tomato, garlic, and olive oil.

QUINOA RISOTTO

This one will have your partner saying, "Ciao, bella!"

1 cup quinoa

1 tablespoon olive oil

1 cup chopped onion

3 cloves garlic, minced

1 cup vegetable broth

1 cup skim milk

8 ounces mushrooms, sliced

¾ cup Parmesan cheese

To remove the bitter outer taste of the quinoa, rinse it several times using a fine-mesh strainer. Heat the olive oil in a saucepan over medium-high heat. Add the onion and cook until soft, stirring constantly. Add the garlic and quinoa, stirring constantly for 1 to 2 minutes. Stir in the broth and milk. Bring to a boil, then reduce heat to low and simmer until the quinoa is tender. Add the mushrooms and cook for another 4 minutes, stirring often. Keep adding more vegetable stock or milk to the quinoa as needed. Remove from heat, sprinkle with cheese, and let stand for a few minutes before serving.

SIMPLY SALMON

This salmon recipe cannot go wrong, and it works famously with a side of brown rice or plain quinoa and a fresh salad.

1–3 tablespoons nonfat or low-fat mayonnaise (enough to cover the salmon)

2 salmon fillets

Pepper

Garlic salt

Seasoning salt

Spread the mayo over the salmon. Cover the fish with the spices to taste. Place on a greased, foil-lined grill at medium-low heat and cook for 30 minutes, or until the salmon is tender. Keep your eye on it, as you don't want it to overcook and dry out.

move it to lose it

In Spanish, the term *la cuarentena* describes the first forty days after you give birth: One day you will feel like you have your body back, and the next day you will wake up feeling four months pregnant again. Your fluctuating body is all part of the adjustment. You have to accept that certain women will regain their pre-baby bodies in a snap. For other women, it could take up to a year or more to get their shape back, which can become intensely frustrating, especially for the divas among us who are not used to being, well, frumpy.

While you may be understandably antsy to get back to your fitness regimen, to ensure adequate healing and recovery try to wait out these forty days before hitting the gym too hard. And even when you are ready to start anew, you must check in with your doctor about which exercises are appropriate and acceptable for your condition—it all depends on your particular birthing experience and your body. It's no fun to look pregnant when you are not, but it will be even less fun to have to endure a prolonged recovery period because you haven't given yourself ample time to restore.

You should wait approximately six weeks before rushing to the abs mat for sit-ups and crunches, because when you are pregnant the abdominal muscles move to the sides, and it does take them some time to shift back into place, a process called diastasis. Be patient: your six-pack can wait. After two months or so, you can start using postpartum belly wraps. (Tauts are fantastic, and you can find them on Brooke Burke's Web site, www.babooshbaby.com.)

Most doctors will likely agree that you should also wait those six weeks before starting (or going back to) a weight-lifting routine. If you hit that forty-day mark and you are just itching to start, remember to begin with low-impact programs (on treadmills or other cardio machines) and work out in small increments of time, starting at fifteen minutes, then twenty, and building on that week to week as your strength returns and your body resettles into itself.

However, caution aside, there are certain things that you can do to kick-start the body's return. I know it seems like I am obsessed with Kegels, and it's true: I cannot say enough about this miracle exercise, which not only helps to reinstate the strength and flexibility of the pelvic floor but also does wonders for the restoration of the vagina. (See "The Super Vagina," page 50, for a refresher on how to do Kegels properly.) Kegels are to pregnancy and birth what scales are to the aspiring pianist: The more you practice, the better you get, and the better you get, the better you will feel.

Other simple exercises you can start early on are leg lifts and pelvic tilts, as well as arm and shoulder exercises using light free weights, which you can keep by the side of your bed for toning before going to sleep and first thing in the morning. Likewise, if you fared well with your prenatal yoga instructor and have come to trust his or her guidance, you can consult your teacher about what exercises and postures are suitable, and slowly work up from there. Patience and perseverance will both play into how well you can do and how far you can go.

Finally, as you wait for things to readjust, consider this a great time to start thinking about your baby's little fitness regimen. It may sound crazy to some, but baby yoga is a great way for you to move around a bit and connect with your baby, while he, too, gets his body moving, blood flowing, and oxygen circulating. There is a great book called *Itsy Bitsy Yoga*, by Helen Garabedian, that is chock-full of postures to help your baby's digestion, sleep, and strength.

mama chic

When your belly sags like an empty sack, your boobs look like torpedoes, and your face resembles that of a bloated panda, eyes all puffed and blackened—perhaps the last word that will come to mind is "glamour." And yet it is precisely this word (and other words like *sexy, flirty,* and *cute*) that might serve you best as a personal mantra as you reconfigure your identity as a woman and attempt to reassert your own sex appeal and femininity. As challenging as it may seem, the road back to hotness does not have to be as bumpy and horrendous as you might expect. But first things first: You *must* honor the time frame. By that I mean that Rome was not built in one day—getting back to your pre-baby gorgeousness can only really happen in its due time.

Chances are you will not want to wear much of anything other than your pajamas for the first few weeks after the birth. It will be like one long pajama party with you and the baby, where you are free to let it all hang out. That, however, does not mean you have to surrender to the frump. *Au contraire*: I definitely recommend splurging on a few sexy robes, or ask for them as baby shower gifts. Japanese-style kimonos, for instance, are colorful and stylish, and you can easily disrobe from them and get yourself to the bathroom, shower, or bed as quickly as needed. Robes, of course, are also ideal for breastfeeding.

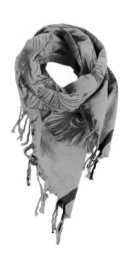
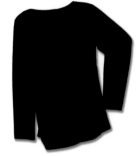

Cashmere shawls, throws, and blankets are also great to indulge in as your body takes its time to recover, giving one the feeling of luxury, comfort, and coziness all at once— and they are also great gifts to request from your friends and family, who will likely be eager to spoil you. But my absolute favorites were big, baggy, loose, cotton dresses that are easy to clean in case of unexpected accidents.

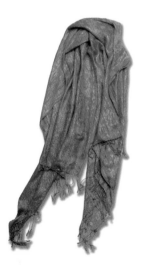
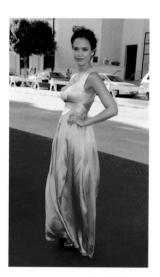

As time passes, you may have to defer to more serious efforts. One of my dearest friends once sent me a set of industrial-strength girdles in the mail. I could not imagine what she wanted me to do with those girdles, and when I called her to inquire, she said, "After you give birth, do yourself a favor and get your ass into that girdle." She explained matter-of-factly, with the wisdom of experience, "You get into that girdle if you ever want to see your old body again." I knew that the girdle would help to remind the muscles of my belly to get back into action again. Fair enough, I thought. Girdle, it is . . . though I did wait the forty days before strapping in.

As the weeks begin to pass, you will likely start to feel more inclined to get out of the robe and back into your jeans. Don't be afraid to keep your maternity clothes around during the transition, and in the process of assembling outfits for yourself each day, try to remain patient and open-minded about what looks good. Remember that looking good is 90 percent about feeling good, so comfort will go a long way during what may seem like an awkward time. Personally, I found that wearing long, flowing dresses in

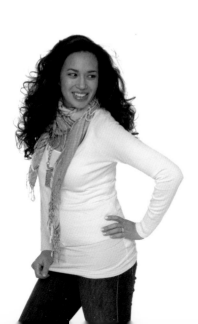
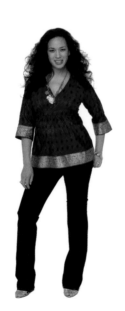
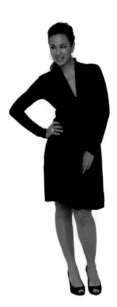

lightweight fabrics gave me the space, ventilation, and easy access for fast maxi pad changes or abrupt trips to the ladies' room. I also found that the darker the color of the dress, the thinner I would feel in it. Since I was breastfeeding and felt incredibly self-conscious about nipple leakage, I realized that wearing patterns was a terrific way to camouflage any unexpected messes.

POST-BABY FASHION TIPS

Here are six of the best no-nonsense tips you'll want to follow:

✳ V-necks make the face and neck look longer and distract attention from any temporary double-chin effect you may be worried about

✳ Avoid dresses or tops that cinch at the waist and opt instead for silhouettes that flare out from beneath the breasts

✳ Now that the bulk of the belly is gone, if you're planning to go out, it's a great time to get back into your high heels (if you feel up to it), as they give a sense of length and instantly sexify any outfit

✳ Long tops in dark colors lengthen the torso and conceal the bulge

✳ An off-the-shoulder top in a baggy silhouette can be at once comfy, sexy, and roomy

✳ Choose bras and panties with extra support and coverage, as you will feel way more comfortable

a little beauty duty never hurt

No matter how much of an effort you may find yourself putting in, there are still postpartum symptoms that are simply beyond our control. Hair loss, or postpartum alopecia, is one such side effect that can drive any woman mad, especially if she's been happily boasting (hormone-induced) luxuriant hair for the last six months. Adult acne may be another pregnancy-related beauty concern, again the product of hormonal chaos in the body, or dark circles, which seem to be inevitable at two hours of sleep per night.

The good news is that there are little things that we can do to cope with these situations. My book, *¡Belleza!: Lessons in Lipgloss and Happiness*, has plenty of quick beauty tips that require minimal effort.

Remember that your diet can significantly help, as foods rich in certain vitamins and minerals are widely known to promote proper hair health. A great way to kick off your day, for example, is to start with a bowl of oatmeal, because oats are loaded with silica, an excellent mineral for the hair. Make it even better for your hair by drizzling a little flax seed oil on it and tossing in a few almonds, as flax seed contains alphalinolenic acid, one of the omega fatty acids, and nuts are packed with zinc, also excellent for hair growth and luster.

Another hair-enhancing snack that's both healthy and easy to make is an avocado wrap: roll up some avocado slices, pumpkin seeds, and brown rice in sheets of seaweed. Seeds of all kinds, actually, are high in B vitamins, as is brown rice, which also happens to be one of the best sources of fiber; the seaweed contains iron, which is also excellent for the hair.

Beyond what you eat, taking high-dosage biotin supplements can help as well. Definitely avoid color treatments and heat-drying your hair. Shampooing hair less often also helps to keep it looking fuller, thicker, and more voluminous.

To treat adult acne, keep the face meticulously clean and toned with a light astringent. Each night before bed, you can dab blemishes with tea tree oil, a wonderful and natural remedy to dry up unsightly pimples. If your case seems severe, consult a dermatologist who may be able to prescribe a more customized skin-care regimen.

To take charge of those dark puffy circles under the eyes, it's time to invest in some no-nonsense eye cream, which you should use in the morning and at night, on a clean face. Also, if you've gone back to drinking coffee, ease up on it, as caffeine is said to worsen the dark circles. Try to nap throughout the day, when your baby is napping, to catch up on rest.

seize the day

If I can leave you with anything other than the advice offered in this book, it is a hearty *congratulations* for making it to the pinnacle of what being a woman is all about: a miraculous realm of femininity that is expressed spiritually and physically, and a dynamic adventure that will unfold for you as one of the most profound lessons of your life. You will see, feel, hear, smell and touch things with a brand new set of senses—those of your child's— and in that magical rediscovery experience the world all over again. Take in the details, savor each moment and watch your little one grow, as you, too, grow exponentially. After all, having a child is almost like a rebirth for you, providing the ultimate impetus to improve yourself physically and mentally, so that you can adequately guide this baby through the world. This is your chance to reinvent your life and maximize the years that come ahead, teaching your little one about love, honesty, gratitude, showing her the beauty and bounty of nature, creating for her a world of joy. So I congratulate you for joining the forces of womanhood and personally welcome you to the fun. Now that you know what pregnancy and birth *really* entail, continue to hold on to the most important tool you can have throughout the entire journey—a *positive attitude*. Love it, own it, and embrace it!

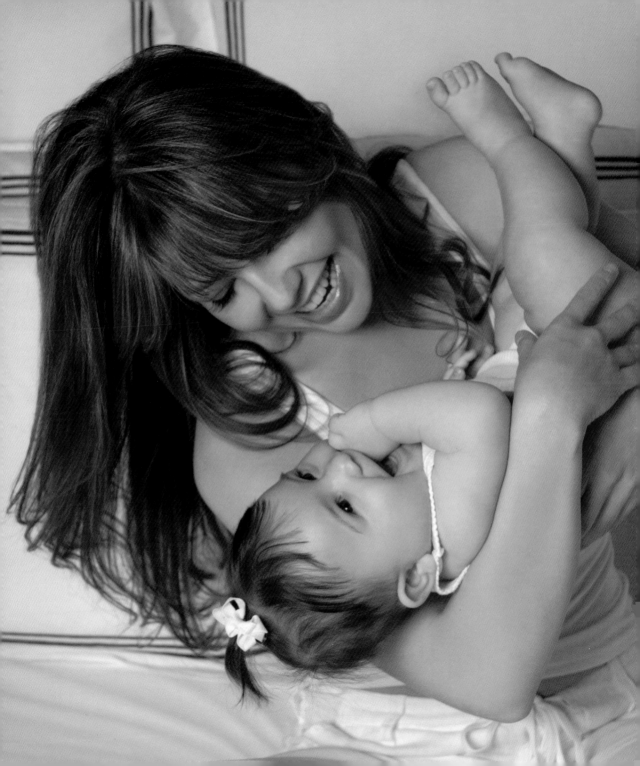

positive affirmations

If you ever need inspiration along the way, take the following affirmations in—daily or weekly, whatever is helpful to you—by keeping them handily posted next to your computer monitor, posted on your fridge, or even include an excerpt as your cell phone's greeting screen. You'll realize that it's a small effort to maintain a big part of your pre and postnatal health: keeping your soul shining and your spirits high . . .

❉ I am beautiful even as I am changing

❉ I am calm and relaxed and my baby feels it

❉ There is nothing to fear

❉ I trust myself to do what is best for my baby

❉ My body is beautiful, capable, and strong

❉ I will have a strong and healthy baby

❉ I am ready to welcome my baby

❉ I trust in my baby

❉ I accept every feeling that accompanies this pregnancy without judgment

❉ My self-love is unconditional

❉ My love for my baby is unconditional

❉ My baby and I are loved and supported

And remember, life is short, so live well, share and laugh.

    With love . . .

    Thalia

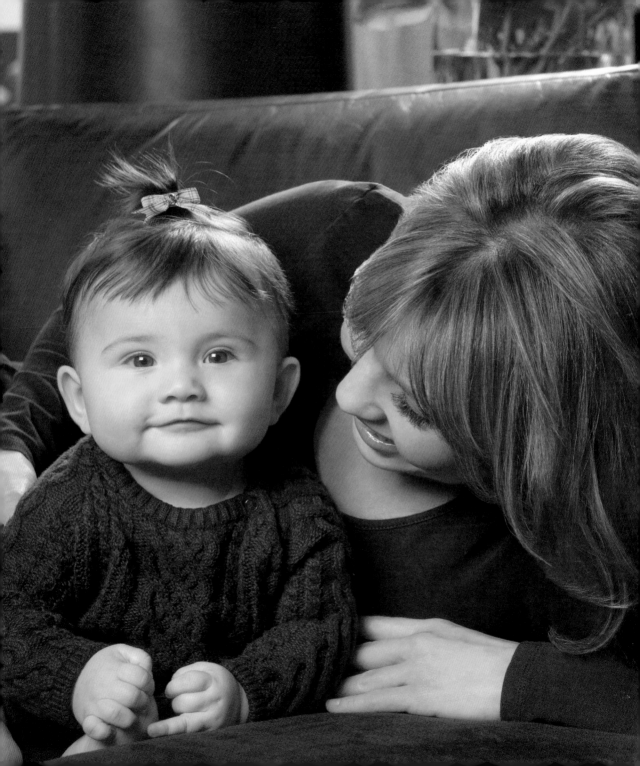

resources

BOOKS

From the Hips: A Comprehensive, Open-minded, Uncensored, and Totally Honest Guide to Pregnancy, Birth and Becoming a Parent by Rebecca Odes and Ceridwen Odes Morris

Healthy Child, Healthy World: Creating a Cleaner, Greener, Safer Home by Christopher Gavigan

Beautiful, Bountiful, Blissful: Experience the Natural Power of Pregnancy and Birth with Kundalini Yoga and Meditation, by Gurmukh Kaur Khalsa, guides you through your pregnancy as a holistic fusion of body, mind, and soul

How to Make a Pregnant Woman Happy: Solving Pregnancy's Most Common Problems—Quickly and Effectively by Uzzi Reiss, MD, and Yfat M. Reiss

What To Expect When You Are Expecting, also known as the bible of pregnancy books, by Heidi Murkoff and Sharm Mazel

The Pregnancy Bible: Your Complete Guide to Pregnancy and Early Parenthood by Joanne Stone, MD, and Keith Eddleman

The Girlfriends' Guide to Pregnancy by Vicki Iovine

What to Expect: Eating Well When You're Expecting by Heidi Murkoff and Sharm Mazel

Ready or Not...Here We Come: The Real Expert's Guide to the First Year with Twins, by Elizabeth Lyons, is both sincere and extremely witty in its account of mothering twins

The Everything Twins, Triplets and More Book: From Seeing the First Sonogram to Coordinating Nap Times and Feedings—All You Need to Enjoy Your Multiples, by Pamela Fierro, is also very complete

Itsy Bitsy Yoga: Poses to Help Your Baby Sleep Longer, Digest Better, and Grow Stronger, by Helen Garabedian, is chock-full of postures to help your baby's digestion, sleep, and strength

Yoga For Pregnancy, Birth and Beyond by Françoise Barbara Freedman and Doriel Hall

Body, Soul, and Baby: A Doctor's Guide to the Complete Pregnancy Experience, from Preconception to Postpartum by Tracey W. Gaudet, MD

I also encourage you to look at my first book, *¡Belleza!: Lessons in Lipgloss and Happiness* for great tips on hair and makeup, the two things you can still totally rock while your pregnant and postpartum body does its thing.

WEB SITES
Fashion/Style Resources for Mama and Baby

www.apeainthepod.com

www.babiesrus.com

www.babooshbaby.com

www.babycenter.com

www.bellydancematernity.com

www.buybuybaby.com

www.dabib.com

www.dayonecenter.com

www.destinationmaternity.com

www.eebee.com

www.elegantbaby.com

www.enfemenino.com/sermadre

www.gap.com
(click on "BabyGap" or "Gap Maternity")

www.giggle.com

www.isabellaoliver.com/maternity-clothes

www.leighluca.com (scarves)

www.lolaetmoi.com

www.lovemybellymaternity.com

www.lucysikes.com

www.milkshop.com

www.momlogic.com

www.motherswork.com

www.mykidscloset.com

www.ouac.com

www.petitetresor.com

www.pumpstation.com

www.sanrio.com (Hello Kitty)

www.spunkysprout.com

www.stokke.com

www.target.com
(click on "Baby" for all pregnancy and birth-related products, including a fantastic line called Liz Lange Maternity for Target)

www.thelittleseed.com

www.tinylove.com

www.upperbreastside.com

www.wendybellissimo.com

www.yummietummie.com

DVDS/MULTIMEDIA

Prenatal Yoga with Shiva Rea, a preeminent yoga instructor known worldwide; and *Yoga Pregnancy* with Heather Seiniger, a certified prenatal yoga teacher and mom

Every Baby's Adventures: www.eebee.com (educational)

BabyFirstTV: www.babyfirsttv.com (educational)

CDS

Zen Garden: The Art of Wellbeing by Colin Willsher

Music for Positive Thinking by Raya Yoga

Living Music by Michael Jones

GENERAL ONLINE RESOURCES

American Medical Association:
www.ama-assn.org

American College of Obstetricians and Gynecologists:
www.acog.org

The Society for Maternal-Fetal Medicine:
www.smfm.org

American College of Nurse-Midwives:
www.acnm.org

International Childbirth Association:
www.icea.org

Women, Infants and Children, a federal agency that assists low-income women:
www.fns.usda.gov/wic/

Medicaid, a federally funded program that helps low-income families and individuals:
www.cms.hhs.gov/home/medicaid.asp

Baby Buggy, an organization that takes donations of baby furniture and equipment:
www.babybuggy.org

acknowledgments

Andrew R. Kramer, MD, Clinical Instructor, Department of Obstetrics, Gynecology, and Reproductive Sciences, The Mount Sinai Hospital, New York, NY

Monica Haim

Barbara Landreth, MD

Giuseppina "Jo-Z" Bonanni

Claudia Nelson, MD

Maria San Jorge, MD

Mona Gabay, MD

Bernard Kruger, MD

Heather Kelly

Lijah Friedman

Joy Bauer MS, RD, CDN

Our models: Expecting Models, New York, Shelley Rapp, Courtenay Driver, Karin Capra, and Rachel Foster

Our production coordinators: Joelle Savino, Christian Martin

Our stylists: David F. Zambrana and Cory Parker, Irma Martinez for Trendy Inc.

Roberto Cavalli: Christiano Mancini

Hair: Joaquin Hortal

Makeup: Sidney Jamila for M·A·C Cosmetics

Our generous product lenders: Mothers Work for Destination Maternity/Mimi Maternity, A Pea in the Pod

Our photo team: Jimmy Ienner Jr., David Gartland

WireImage and Getty Images

Carnegie Hill Imaging for Women, Dr. Andrei Rebarber

To everyone at Chronicle Books on my team: Jodi Warshaw, Aya Akazawa, Carleigh Bell, River Jukes-Hudson, Molly Glover, Molly Jones, Yolanda Accinelli

Joanne Oriti

Nora Jacobs

Mariela Perez

And, of course, Tommy Mottola, Yolanda Miranda, my friends, my family, and my loyal loving fans

...and my ONE AND ONLY TRUE INSPIRATION FOR THIS BOOK, SABRINA SAKAË...THIS IS FOR YOU!

photo credits

index